21 Days of Simple Changes

—

Supercharge Your Vitality
for Our High-Velocity World

Gregory Florez

ISBN-13:978-1502557780
ISBN-10:1502557789

Acknowledgements

I am grateful that you picked up this book and hope that you find it useful.

This was my first book. It was hard. Thankfully, I had so much support and help.

First and foremost I'd like to thank my editor Laura Lawson. She was sent to me by angels and she certainly proved to be one herself. She helped me concentrate. She read numerous versions of the manuscript and every suggestion she made was flawless. This book would not have been written without her. Period. Thank you from the bottom of my heart.

Also helping me with so many valuable details were Brenda Fogg and Stephanie Ashmore, MS, RD, CD. You handled so much of the detail work that needed doing, and both of you exceeded any expectations I had (including tight deadlines).

Thanks, also to some of my colleagues and mentors over the years who made me want to write a book: Dr. Cedric X Bryant, Kevin McCarthy M.S., and Richard Cotton, M.S. You all in your own way have contributed to my education and helped plant the seeds that became this book.

Lastly, thank you to my wife and partner for life, Kerry, for being patient with me and always encouraging me when I thought I couldn't do it (and deleted yet another manuscript). More than anything you have always believed in me even when I didn't. It has made all of the difference. I love you forever.

Contents

21 Days of Simple Changes

—

*Supercharge Your Vitality
for Our High-Velocity World*

Preface

Not long ago, or far away there was a culture of people on this planet who had time and energy for their families, extended families, and friends. When they closed the door at work or on a project (literally and figuratively) they had the energy and vitality to transition to a focus on their family and community. But that was before the age of information, technology, "Big Data" and of course even before the Internet. Now, more than likely, you rush from one thing to the other, constantly trying to multi—task, being pulled in many different directions. You might be unfocused and lack vitality for yourself or those who are most important to you.

Well, it's time to claim your vitality once again and I hope to help you do just that in this book. *21 Days of Simple Changes* is a compilation of some of the most important changes that my clients have made in my more than 27 years in the vitality coaching business. I am so very grateful to these clients. They have taught me more about myself and vitality than I ever thought possible. Thanks to them from the bottom of my heart. Bless you.

My greatest wish for you is more physical and mental vigor no matter your age or current situation. Thanks for reading!

Gregory Florez

Part 1

Make Simple Changes for 21 Days

The Bottom Line

If you are like most of my clients your life has become one long list of things that must be done—often now! In many cases our lives have become so filled with other *obligations* that our own vitality takes a back seat to nearly everything else. But if you increase your own vitality, that will help you to complete important tasks on time and give you the energy to deal with important decisions surrounding how you spend your entire life.

Time is not finite, but energy and vitality are. I'm grateful that you have picked up this book given how utterly busy you probably are. Trust me—it's a great start. And getting started is the most important step in beginning to reclaim your vitality. This book will help you start small and build successful habits in 21-day increments. In this way you will not only help your body but also begin to train your mind to be more agile.

What does vitality mean to *you*?

Is it having more energy? Sleeping better? Slimming down? Having better concentration at work, preventing disease? As you begin to read this book it is crucial to define what becoming more vital means to you and *own* it for yourself.

Remember that vitality is your natural state of being and that you *deserve* to be vital. Also remember that vitality is personal to each of us. The worst thing you can do is to define vitality in the way that a public figure, or even a good friend, does. Also, starting a vitality program because your spouse, partner, or even physician tells you so will generally not work in the long term. Your *personal* motivation and level of that motivation will keep you going when you are ready. And your picking up this book tells me that you are ready.

Using this Book

The 70 Simple Changes here are numbered for convenience, but that doesn't mean you need to read from cover to cover. In fact, I encourage you to browse the book and mark the simple changes that are most relevant and important to you. You can always come back to others when you need them. You will probably, however, want to take a look at the Reaching Your Goals Worksheet in Appendix 1 sooner vs. later (more below). This worksheet will help guide your efforts on the Simple Changes you want to make. So feel free to open this book to any page or section at any time. I'm betting your intuition will take you to the right page more times than not. Remember to use the tools in the Appendixes—more than once if you need to. And always remember that if you lose your focus on your Simple Changes you just need to start again. Remember, it's simple!

If you have a goal but need help choosing Simple Changes to reach the goal, look at Appendix 2, *Simple Changes for Specific Goals*. There you'll find commonly sought goals and changes to achieve them.

Another good way to start is to look at the first five Simple Changes in the next section—the ones I call the 5 Quick-Start Changes. Of all the Simple Changes I've developed or seen, these are the ones that have been most fundamental for increasing the vitality of my clients, and myself!

Begin with 3 Simple Changes for 21 Days

Short-term Simple Changes lead to long term, lasting changes that are more likely to stick. That's why I urge you to focus on only a few Simple Changes at first.

To succeed, begin with no more than 3 Simple Changes for the first 21 days

This is what I have found to be the "sweet spot" for most people— the approach that yields the most success, is easy to do, and leaves you ready for more. Remember that it takes about 21 days for a habit to form. After the first 21 days, assess where you are and decide whether you want to change your focus, add a new Simple Change, or stick with the current plan. If you stick with Simple Changes you can see much greater personal change in as little as 4 to 6 weeks!

Some additional things to keep in mind as you strive to become more vital through Simple Changes:

- Schedule your vitality rituals early in the week—every week.
- If you get sidetracked do not dwell on this. Get started right back the next day.
- Life will occasionally interrupt you (sick family members, impossible work deadlines, etc). Know that going in and have a plan for getting right back on track when other priorities come up.

Building your personal vitality is a very important step that warrants you sitting down—with paper and pen and thinking it through. Don't worry, I've supplied the form in Appendix 1. There you'll see an outline for your personal vitality plan, the *Reaching Your Goals* worksheet. You can either begin to fill out the worksheet now, save it for last, or even begin to populate the form as you read. Take some reflective time to think about how you want to proceed as you go through the *Reaching Your Goals* worksheet. Completing this exercise will help inform how you use this book as a guide to a more vital you.

Let's begin....

Part 2

70 Simple Changes

The 5 Quick-Start Changes

If I could recommend only five Simple Changes to increase your vitality, these would be the ones. They have been fundamental for so many of my clients—and for me, personally. So if you're looking for an immediate beginning to your vitality plan, start here!

1. Hydrate!

I'll begin with perhaps the easiest Simple Change that exists—drinking more water. Every day the average adult will lose about 10 cups of water just by normal body functions including breathing and sweating. (1)

Being dehydrated causes many unhealthy side effects including:

- Headaches
- Inability to focus
- Dry mouth and skin
- Poor bowel movements
- Weight gain
- Irritability.

Long term, dehydration can affect circulatory function, blood sugar, and a host of other lifestyle-related diseases. Proper hydration is also an important part of losing weight and maintaining a healthy weight. Often when our brain first gives us a hunger signal it really wants hydration. If you feel "hungry" and drink 12 to 16 ounces of water, then wait 10 minutes, you'll often find that your hunger has disappeared or diminished.

On the other hand, healthy hydration can bring some important benefits including:

- Fewer headaches
- Healthier skin
- More energy throughout the day
- Help with weight management
- Improved bowel function.

So how much is enough? Experts suggest a daily intake of 91 ounces (2.7 liters) for women and 125 ounces (3.7 liters) for men, depending upon activity level, body size, and perspiration/activity rate. (2) In a high-velocity lifestyle it can be very hard to remember to drink during the day.

Here's a tip: Keep a water bottle at your desk, in your car, near your nightstand—essentially anywhere that you will remember to drink. Out of sight means out of mind. Put post-it notes in strategic places or even alarms on your smart phone or computer to remind you to drink. If the experts' recommendations seem like a lot, consider this: We are awake around 18 hours a day. 64 ounces is about 2 sips of water per waking hour. Almost anyone can commit to that amount.

Start today and commit for 21 days.

2. Have Water and Healthy Food at Hand

If you're like most of us you live in a state of perpetual motion, whether you work for a living or not. We are very likely running to meetings, errands, classes, etc. in a "just in time" manner. When this happens we often forget to eat or drink water and get too hungry, too tired, and too thirsty. Worse yet, we reach for anything that looks like food including the receptionist's M&Ms jar, or a piece of someone's birthday cake.

To counter that unhealthy "reach," *always be prepared.* Here's what works for most of my clients: before the week begins buy fruit, bottled water, trail mix, nuts, healthy energy bars and other high quality snacks. Always have them near you. The reason I say before the week begins is that once it does you are off and running! Look at your routine to figure out where to put the snacks. It may be that these are kept in a desk drawer, your briefcase, car and *anywhere* you spend time.

3. 10 minutes of exercise counts

The U.S. Department of Health and Human Services recommends 150 minutes of moderate-intensity aerobic activity per week for major health benefits, commonly promoted as 30 minutes 5 times a week (3). Research has found that you can get the same benefits whether you work out all at once or in small bouts throughout the day (4). In other words, you can plan your day with breaks of no more than 10 minutes x 3 to:

- Take a brisk walk
- Do several body weight exercises, e.g. push-ups, sit-ups, etc.
- Use a work break to stretch or climb stairs
- Get outside and do any type of exercise
- Use time waiting for a meal to cook to perform some strength exercises, or even Yoga movements
- Use bands or dumbbells strategically located in places where you'll use them.

In other words, it all adds up if you can get to 30 minutes. Particularly in the first 21 days, schedule even 10 minute bouts of exercise and make sure you have ways that will remind you to do them throughout your day.

4. Learn To Breathe Deeply

Most of us use only a portion of our lung capacity because we breathe so shallowly on a daily basis. Breathing deeply is associated with so many benefits including:

- Better relaxation and healthier sleep
- More energy
- The ability to calm yourself before or following a stressful event
- Better oxygen and blood flow through our entire system
- Increased mindfulness and concentration.

Most of us have breathed in a shallow fashion our whole lives. Our lungs do not end at the top of our rib cage but rather extend down to near our belly. Take a moment to use greater lung capacity. Breathe in slowly through your nose for a count of six. Next, breathe out for a count of 8 to completely empty your lungs. Repeat 7 more times and notice the difference in relaxation and perhaps calmness that you feel. Try it now, if you please. Once you learn this technique you will be amazed at how many applications it has in your life—all of them positive. It takes some practice but once you have mastered it, you will have it as a tool forever. In Appendix 3, Resources to Help with Your Simple Changes, are some resources including apps that I like and use to get you started. And start you should . . . today.

5. Meditate for even 5 Minutes a Day

This might be the most important tip that I can give you. It has been so for a multitude of my clients. Meditating has so many scientifically proven benefits including:

- Lowered blood pressure
- Lowered cholesterol
- Improved energy
- A better, more "grounded" mood
- Less agitation

- Greater mental clarity
- More even temper, mindfulness, and *presence*
- Improved sleep.

First of all meditation does not have to be a deep, mystical, time-consuming ritual. In fact, it is among the simplest yet most powerful tools you can use toward your personal vitality. Meditation can be accomplished through a variety of methods but in keeping with my Simple Changes philosophy, I'll share what I believe to be the most practical and easiest way to get started. If you are so inclined, I've provided several resources in Appendix 3 for you.

Meditation—unlike what many people believe—is not about making your mind free of all clutter. Rather it is about sitting still and simply observing your breath and mind and all of its voices and mostly useless bantering. In fact Jack Kornfield, noted American Buddhist Priest and author of several books, says it best—and I paraphrase here—"Our minds are like untrained puppies that frolic all over the place, and meditation helps us to see that." Here is the simplest meditation I know for busy people to start on.

1. Find a place that is quiet in your home or office and have a cushion or even a straight-backed chair to sit on so that you are comfortable.
2. Commit to sit for at least 5-10 minutes.
3. Sit tall with your legs crossed (or with feet firmly planted on the floor if you are seated in a chair) and your eyes closed or fixed on an object about 2 feet in front of you using a "soft" gaze.
4. Begin to breathe in and out and let your breath gradually slow and deepen.
5. Count your breaths (I suggest to count in multiples of 8 breathes, then start over. You can use whatever works for you however).
6. When your mind wanders to any thought simply notice it. DO NOT try to change or tame each thought but rather bring it to your attention then go back to counting your breaths.

7. Repeat. Every day. It can help to do this at the same time of the day if possible.

8. Do this for 21 days and I'm willing to bet you will notice a difference.

Meditation has been around for centuries and is practiced by most of my clients including many of the busiest people I've ever known. Anyone can find 5-10 minutes each day for this simple and powerful practice.

65 More Simple Changes

So those are the 5 Quick-Start changes. But not every Simple Change is right for every person, and you need to choose the ones that work for you. Here are 65 more changes that are just as simple and easy to help you build your own vitality.

6. Get Off "Automatic Pilot"

Warning: this is a tough one. Old habits—actually even newer ones—can be hard to break. You may have habits like that you want to quit, but you can't break the inertia keeping you in them. It's particularly hard when there is some gratification associated with the habit, e.g., "This donut always tastes good for breakfast in the morning. I will have one." Instead of deciding, "I'm going to stop my donut habit completely starting right now," think about having a donut two fewer days out of the week to start with, as a Simple Change for the first 21 days. From there it will be easier to transition to more days of replacing donuts with an energizing breakfast.

Remember to leave yourself cues or reminders to help you along the way—alarms in your phone or a note on your schedule.

7. Make Your Exercise Intense

In exercise, intensity rules. Period. Whether you are looking to get stronger, increase endurance, or become more flexible. Now this doesn't mean you need to start out by running wind sprints, or lift weights like an Olympic athlete. What it *does* mean is that you need to fatigue your body by doing things like using the interval program on cardiovascular equipment, or performing strength exercises to *fatigue*. This intensity can be less than comfortable, but it will keep pushing your body to becoming more supple, stronger, and also strengthening all of your systems.

Here's an example: Say you are currently using the elliptical trainer. You perform a 5 to 7 minute warm-up followed by walking, jogging, or stepping at a pre-determined pace for 30 minutes. Although you are certainly doing your body good, you are going to stop progressing at a certain point. Better that you:

- Use the interval program on a cardiovascular machine
- Try a different flexibility routine
- Make sure you perform your strength exercises to *fatigue* by gradually adding resistance as your body can handle it.

This is perhaps the most beneficial tip I can give you if you want to see gains. It also might mean that because you are exercising with more intensity, you won't have to exercise as long as you have been. Start mixing it up and add intensity.

8. Prepare Your Eating Plan *before* the Week Begins

For most of us, our weeks are packed, whether we work for a living or run a household. This generally means—sadly—that once the week begins we're already playing catch-up. Nutrition is such a valuable part of a complete vitality program. On the weekend, plan what you will eat for breakfasts, snacks, and dinners and go shopping for those things *before* Monday morning. Keep the healthy foods front and center (out of sight is out of mind) whether it be in your refrigerator, desk, or even snacks in your car once the week begins. In this way you will be much more likely to reach for the healthy choices when things become hectic during the week. If you need extra motivation remember that eating well:

- Stabilizes your energy throughout the day
- Helps you lose and manage your weight
- Improves your mood and ability to engage with others
- Decreases risks of many diseases
- Improves your sleep patterns
- Sharpens your focus.

Start this ritual next weekend. It is one of the simplest and highest value Simple Changes!

9. Have Recovery Time for Every Stressor

Two researchers at the turn of the 20th Century, John Dillingham Dodson and Robert Yerkes, did studies that show the following: Stress is good...to a certain point.(5) The scientists found that our bodies create more epinephrine, cortisol, and other chemicals in order to prepare ourselves for many upcoming events. Getting ready for a meeting, anticipating meeting someone for the first time, and preparing for an exam are but a few examples of stress. At best, we peak in our stress at a level that is appropriate to the event. However, every stressor must have recovery following it in equal measure. There is a diagram for this phenomenon in Appendix 4.

The problem is that for millions of us our stress continues unabated for long periods of time without recovery. If we don't get recovery on a regular basis very bad things can happen from strokes, to heart attacks, high blood pressure, depression and a multitude of other diseases. In a society that is "always on" we badly need to change the paradigm from stress to recovery. Since it doesn't look like we'll slow down anytime soon it is up to you to build in periods of recovery, whether you work for a living, have children at home that need to be cared for, or simply have a hectic life.

The lack of recovery is possibly the most common ailment that I find with my clients on a daily basis. Unfortunately, I've witnessed the fallout from continued stress with many of them.

In addition to health issues, it is important to build in breaks or recovery time between periods of work. This recovery period yields many benefits: It ensures that you will stay fresh and do quality work throughout a project or task. Recovery time will keep your mind stimulated to possibly come up with more creative or better solutions.

Learn what recovery means for you and take back even small bits of time in recovery rituals whenever you can. Recovery can be anything that takes you off of the roller coaster of repeated stress, including:

- Listening to music
- Exercising
- Meditating
- Going for a short walk
- Seeing a movie or play
- Watching your kids at play
- Taking a power nap.

Even 15 minutes of doing something pleasurable that breaks the stress cycle can be very helpful—and in some cases your health depends upon it.

10. Build in Recovery Time from Work to Home

In our over-programmed, time starved society the time we have to "breathe out" is often limited or lacking all together. We all need recovery time, particularly when transitioning from one task to the next. An example of this transition is working hard all day and going from work to being at home with your partner and children. Many studies point to everything from insomnia, to heightened anxiety and high blood pressure when we feel the stress of not getting proper recovery time. (6)

Make recovery time a priority. Here is an example of what many of our clients do to make the transition from work to home: listen to music or a book on tape on the commute home. Close to home, stop for a minute and do a series of "letting go" deep breathes to calm yourself and make the mental switch to home. Doing this will make you much more present for yourself and your family. Some of the psycho-physiological benefits of recovery time include:

- Breaking the elevating stress cycle
- Allowing the brain to flush waste and clear out precious space
- Reducing anxiety, agitation, even depression
- Making you more present for the people you most care about.

11. Develop A Bedtime Ritual

Trouble falling asleep, awakening often, tiredness throughout the day are just a few of the symptoms of poor sleeping habits. The long term symptoms are far more revealing. A few examples:

- A new American study showed that even one night of bad sleep causes changes equivalent to a blow to the head! This study goes on to say that subjects had an increased risk of Alzheimer's, Parkinson's disease, and even Multiple Sclerosis. (7)

- Other studies show that there is a cognitive decline in the ability to function during the day associated with lack of enough sleep. This means that you are less able to think clearly and are more forgetful. (8)

Sleep deprivation is now considered a national epidemic by the National Sleep Foundation. Over 60% of adult Americans live with some type of sleep problem from insomnia, to not getting enough sleep, to waking repeatedly during the night. (9) That means 6 out of 10 of you reading this book right now are sleep-deprived! Work, technology, family issues, and even worry about the future of the planet have all conspired to give so many of us less sleep than we need.

A bit of science behind restful sleep is in order here. Science now shows us that restful sleep helps flush out waste from our brains and actually helps create new synaptic connections during the night. (10) In addition it takes newly gained information and learning and helps synthesize it and process it. Know this: even while sleeping the brain never rests. It is quietly and efficiently processing thoughts and data from the day and helping to make them relevant.

Sleep deprivation is not always easy to cure, but one very helpful Simple Change is to develop a bedtime ritual. This means doing something very different than frantically checking e-mail (or wasting sleep time on Facebook), rushing to get the kids to bed, or cramming for a work project due the next day. Also, watching the news can be troubling for some, with all of the negativity and real life issues going on around the globe. And if that isn't enough there is new, compelling research that shows that looking at a blue light (computers, tablets) before bed triggers a response in the brain that essentially acts as a stimulant, preventing sleep. (11)

Many of us have gotten by on 5 to 6 hours of sleep per night for a long time. This does not mean it is a healthy practice. Almost all of the research shows that we need between 7 to 9 hours of quality sleep in order to be alert, refreshed and better able to function at anything during the day.

So, at least 30 minutes before bed begin to wind down with a ritual that tells your mind and body that it is time for sleep. Some of my clients' tried and true rituals include:

- Taking a hot bath or long shower
- Reading to your child
- Reading for pleasure yourself
- Stretching
- Meditation, prayer, or a breathing ritual

A bedtime routine is essential. Sweet dreams.

12. Keep a Food Journal—a Short One

I'm generally not a big fan of keeping copious, long-term notes on what you put in your body. It often takes a lot of work and if you miss a day it gives you a good reason to stop doing it (by beating yourself up). That said, a Kaiser Permanente Center for Health Research study found that participants lost significantly more weight when keeping a food journal! (12) Keeping a journal makes you accountable for your food choices. You may catch your-self sneaking more empty calories throughout the day than you are aware of. You may scan the food log at the end of the day to realize you did not have any vegetables and think of how to rem-edy this for the next day. Taking a moment to record what you eat also provides you with the opportunity to consider why you are eating. Are you really hungry or are you reaching for something out of habit?

So the Simple Change I suggest is to keep a brief *recall* food log, which helps you look at what you've actually eaten in the past 2 to 3 days (vs. looking forward). This tends to be an "honest" assessment, and looking forward has the effect of making you eat better because you know you'll be writing it down!

Doing it in arrears also provides an accurate accounting of what your daily intake is really made up of. Remember to write down everything that goes into your mouth—even say the amount of cream (estimated) in your coffee.

From here you can essentially become your own dietitian. Simply scan the record and look for the foods that are providing "empty" calories. For example:

- Candy of any type
- Café Latte's filled with sugar and syrups
- Additives, including sugar (honey, agave, glucose, fructose), flavorings, sauces, etc.
- Overly large portions in a meal
- Eating late in the evening or snacking in the middle of the night

If you want to become more serious about this, and likely you may; I've provided a list of some of my favorite dietary apps in Appendix 3, Resources to Help You with Simple Changes. These apps will help you record your intake.

It's important to know what *really* goes into your body vs. what you are telling yourself is on a regular basis. In this way you can start making Simple Changes to the way you eat going forward. This will help you eat mindfully making weight and energy management simple and possible.

13. Practice Mindfulness

This is where you can really make some changes, starting today. We are so overwrought and flooded with technology and information that more, and more are we unaware of the impact we have when we actually *speak* to each other—vs. sending a text, e-mail, etc.

Being mindful starts with a decision to "be present in the moment." Meditation—as mentioned earlier—is helpful. But you can also simply stop, notice that you have too much on your mind, and make a decision to be present in that *very moment*. Being present can mean listening *fully* to a conversation, playing with your child, even cooking.

Being mindful can be a huge asset whether you work or spend time with friends and family. Are you constantly ruminating on what you should be doing? Thinking about a work project? Constantly scanning your smart phone, Facebook, or e-mail? Make no mistake; the times in which we live make it very difficult for us to concentrate on one thing at a time. It takes a decision to listen—to yourself and others—and a commitment to mindfulness.

Mindfulness is not esoteric or mystical at all. It simply means to be present in the moment as many times per day as you can. Make that decision and then use tools to help you, like:

- Breathing and meditation
- Turning on alarms in your phone to remind you of stop and be mindful
- Turning off all media (once you've reminded yourself!)
- Making a decision to "be here now"
- Breathing and staying in the moment for as long as you can
- Repeat

I promise that you will find any relationship, including the one with yourself, will be enriched. You will also likely come up with new insights, and be more calm and centered in your life. Being mindful in the society in which we live is not easy. Try some of the techniques above or useful apps for breathing in Appendix 3 to help you, and personalize them for yourself. You will be amazed at what comes up for you and how you process information.

14. Take at least three Walking Meetings per Week

Technology and information overload keep us tethered to our desks for much more time than is healthy for us. In fact, the clients I work with would stay at their desks for 12 hours every day without taking so much as a lunch break if possible (and sometimes, sadly, it is!). Sitting for long periods of time is associated with poor posture, high blood pressure, and even coronary disease. (13) (14) Schedule and take 10 minute walking meetings *outside,* three times per week as a start. These meetings will help give your brain a rest, give your muscles and body some movement, and even help generate creative thought. You will get more natural light (and even some Vitamin D depending upon the conditions), give your body and mind a break, and likely be more present with your co-workers, clients—even family members.

I realize that in many cases this is a pretty dramatic departure from the norm. If you don't feel comfortable doing this, talk with your boss—or peers—and let them know what you are doing and why. As with other Simple Changes this will take some time to un-tether yourself from your technology and desk. Make it a priority by scheduling it and committing to do it. Again, I can't stress enough how important it is to let others know you are doing this to increase the vitality—and gain support—of all parties concerned.

I generally recommend *not* taking your phone—you can do without it for 10 minutes. However, if the meeting will have some action items, buy a small handheld recorder and use it to log important items.

15. Pick Up A Pen

Remember that vitality includes exuberance of mind as well as body. It seems like texting has become as easy as breathing these days. How often do you pop off a quick thank you text or e-mail to someone you want to recognize? Pretty easy, and in these times, pretty ubiqui-tous. I'll bet that even as you read this there is someone in your life that you'd like to reach out to—to thank or just let them know you are thinking of them—and plan on doing so with a text.

Instead, how about writing out a simple but heartfelt letter or note? A good way to get into the habit of doing this is to keep some note-cards handy. Then, when the urge arises take five minutes to write to that person, using pen and paper. You'll be amazed at how this will help you take a break, maybe smile, and improve your mental state. Taking this writing break sends chemicals to your brain that can help ward off negative or even hopeless thoughts in some cases. Moreover, sending a written note sends a message that you care enough to take the time, and also helps strengthen relationships, both personally and professionally. Finally, writing can help you clarify your thoughts and even help discover and discard negative ones.

16. Work with a Personal Trainer

We are surrounded by programs and promises for "ripped abs" and quick weight loss every day—sometimes often during the day. Here are questions for anyone reading this who has tried a 30-day or 6-week program over a year ago. Did it stick? Have you kept the weight off and is the routine, well, routine? Almost all of my clients have answered "no" to the above.

The fact is that you didn't get out of shape in a month, and it's highly unlikely that you'll get back into great shape in the same amount of time. No matter what anyone tells you any worthwhile fitness routine has the following components:

- Cardiovascular exercise
- Strength training
- Flexibility training
- Sensible nutrition

Now, it is possible to see physical changes within a month to 6 weeks but highly unlikely a complete transformation. Here's a Simple Change: start with an expert. Hire a Certified Personal Trainer to at least help you get started. Someone who is qualified will help you paint a picture of complete health and get you on the road to total fitness. He or she will also be able to help you whether you belong to a gym or have little to no equipment at home. Moreover the trainer will "meet you where you live" in terms of your current fitness without the risk of overdoing or injury.

To help find a trainer, there are many great resources out there including word of mouth. My favorite place to find a qualified trainer is through The American Council on Exercises: www.acefitness. org/ace-fit/locate-trainer/.

17. Schedule Your Priorities

Steven Covey, the author of one of the best-selling books of all time, *The Seven Habits of Highly Effective People,* states, (15) "The key is not to prioritize what's on your schedule, but to schedule your priorities." Nothing could be closer to the truth. Chances are that, whether you work for a living or not, your life is full of obligations. From ferrying children to soccer games to helping sick relatives there seems to be no "white space" in your calendar for you to attend to your own highest priorities. And guess what? There won't be unless you make some.

I have my clients schedule vital activities in three-month periods. Going much longer than that usually means major course corrections. Any less, and vital activities tend to slip away. Sit down at the beginning of a quarter and realistically schedule in activities like exercise, meditation, at-home meals, etc. I know a schedule might sound rigid but creating it will force you to truly become vital in the long run. If you're like many people, after a few quarters this will become natural to you.

18. Do Your Work in Chunks

The human brain is wired to concentrate fully for between 60 and 90 minutes. (16) It is at this point that your concentration—and possibly quality of work—begins to decline. We are so conditioned to get massive amounts of work done that we plow forward, with the consequences of more mistakes and diminishing quality. This grinding focus also causes us to forget to eat, become cranky, and even work through periods of time when we are sleepy (dramatically increasing the chance for mistakes).

It's time to make time for breaks. Every day. At least every 90 minutes. Taking breaks will require re-training your body and your mind, so start small. Put an alarm on your smart-phone or computer that reminds you to take a five minute break *at least* every hour and a half. Use this time to get up from your desk, walk around, possibly get a small snack or if it's early in the day, a cup of coffee. The act of merely taking any kind of break will leave you refreshed and ready to re-engage in your work. Taking even a 10 minute break can spark your creativity, or help you break through a problem you have been noodling on. So set an alarm or leave yourself a note in your planner or schedule for at least the first 3 weeks.

Remember that as humans we are designed to work in "chunks" of time. Swimming against this tide will simply cause more anxiety and lessen the quality of your work.

19. Have Fun—Even A Little

Many experts and best-selling books observe that our lives have become so frantic that we've forgotten to have fun in the moment. Think of yourself and your life: How often do you smile or laugh? Is it less than before you worked so hard or had kids and more responsibilities? Does your workplace provide an environment where there is some levity, or laughter in meetings or in one on one time?

If not it's time to re-write the rules. Smile and have some fun each day. If you need something to jump-start this Simple Change, start reading the jokes that you get from that "annoying" friend who sends them. (You know, the ones you delete because you have a zillion e-mails to read.) Read the comics *at work!* Spend break time with the man or woman in Accounting who always makes everyone in the office laugh.

At home make up a zany—even messy—project and do it with your kids. Do so without worrying about the clean-up or mess that it makes. Be in the moment with them. Fun time with them is so precious and fleeting. Remind yourself of that when the red paint spills on your carpet!

Having fun is serious business that will help your mood, possibly lower your blood pressure, and bring back the missing laughter in your life.

20. Do One Big Thing Daily

I understand that you are overwhelmed with work, family, extended family, and friend's commitments. I suppose that we all are. Keep making lists and cross of what you can but at the very least prioritize *one big thing* to get done every day. Put it at the top of your list or in the highest priority category. Get it done in the first part of the day when your body and mind are at their freshest. This Simple Change can have a huge effect on your day, and your life if you start doing this regularly. Start now.

Listen, if you really look at those to-do lists you'll soon realize that you only generally get them partially done anyway. And know that the "overwhelm" will probably always be there in the times in which we live. Make peace with it. Heck, even embrace it knowing that although it will never go away, it will begin to occupy a much smaller space in the back of your mind.

21. **Make Fitness a Priority**

Some of the benefits of even a basic fitness program include:

- Increased energy
- Improved metabolic function (burn more calories)
- Decrease in your resting heart rate, cholesterol
- Sharpened memory
- Greater chance of longevity
- More mobility for all daily activities

There are so many reasons to make fitness something that you schedule and accomplish in your daily/weekly routine. Remember that a fitness program does not have to be a long and involved process. Just getting moving will help immeasurably! The key is in scheduling your routine and keeping appointments for fitness with the same diligence as you do other activities. Doing so will make all of your other activities richer and more carefree.

22. **Get Inexpensive Exercise Equipment for Travel**

Often, the biggest saboteur of a well-intended exercise program is travel—for business or for pleasure. Missing your routine for several days can sidetrack you on the road to better health. On the other hand purchasing and *using* inexpensive exercise equipment can help you:

- Squeeze in a 10-minute workout—anytime, anywhere
- Keep your equipment close at hand rather than taking up a large space in your home (or carry-on).
- Keep portable equipment in your office, car, and carry-on so that you won't miss a workout
- Ultimately ensure that you get at least 10 minutes of a workout each day
- Keep your string of scheduled workouts intact!

Dozens of companies make portable equipment, from folding, packable exercise mats, to rubberized strength training tubing and stretch bands. They are inexpensive. Buy some. Keep them in your primary carry-on luggage at all times. Have a simple and quick "default" program that you can accomplish on the road. Also pack a good pair of walking or exercise shoes and if not a workout outfit, at least some loose fitting clothing. Use these tools.

Remember that being on the road does not mean you have to abandon your exercise program entirely. You also don't have to execute a complete program. Think of maintenance as your goal. Appendix 5 gives the FitAdvisor Road Warrior Card Exercises for Simple Changes. In these exercises, I have a suggested strength training routine using rubber tubing that can take less than 15 minutes.

One final note: Ten minutes of quality exercise counts. If schedule or travel makes it such that you don't have time for a longer routine, pick something you can do in ten minutes—perhaps broken up in two or three chunks per day. You will be much more likely to return to your regular routine if you do this.

23. Eat Fruits or Vegetables before Eating Out

Often, eating out is an inevitable part of our daily lives. You know that you are often limited in your choices of foods at a group or business dinner. So eat a small salad, or a piece of whole fruit about a half an hour before going out. This Simple Change will increase your fluid intake—making you feel more full—and add fiber, also making you feel fuller. Once you make this change a habit you might amaze yourself at how much less you eat at dinner. You'll feel better about yourself and consume fewer calories—and maybe even less alcohol, too.

24. **Alternate Water with Alcoholic Beverages**

Speaking of alcohol and hydration.... Here is a trick that one of my clients swears by: When you are out and consuming alcoholic beverages (generally high in sugars and poor quality calories) drink one 12 to 16 ounce glass of water in between each alcoholic drink. This pattern will help you to drink less alcohol, keep you hydrated, and ensure that you will feel better the next morning! You'll also likely eat less of the higher calorie hors d' oeuvres and snacks that are available, and maybe be more sensible about dessert.

Generally speaking the alcoholic beverages that contain the most sugars and/or empty calories include:

- Margarita
- Daiquiri
- Pina Colada
- Bailey's Irish Cream
- Other drinks with sugar evident in them
- Most mixed drinks

Try to stick to red wine if possible. It is filled with antioxidants and provides much more nutritional value per drink.

25. **Eat the Good Fats**

Okay, I'm asking you to trust me here (or look up the latest research)....Fats are good! They are a healthy part of a balanced diet. The tricky part is knowing which fats to limit or avoid. Fat provides a terrific source of energy as well as a great depot for storing it. It is an important part of cell membranes, helping govern what gets into cells and what comes out. The body uses cholesterol as the starting point to make estrogen, testosterone, vitamin D, and other vital compounds. Fats are also biologically active molecules that can influence how muscles respond; different types of fats can also fire up or cool down inflammation.

Often people will switch to low-fat or fat-free items when trying to lose weight or eat healthier. But this approach can be hazardous:

- Many reduced and low fat items replace the missing fat with sugar to maintain texture and flavor. The added sugar often makes up for the calories from the "missing" fat. Too many added sugars can also have a negative impact on your blood lipid profile (cholesterol and triglycerides) and have serious long-term health effects.

- Some fats are essential: Your body cannot produce them on its own and needs them from your diet. In this group are Omega-3 fatty acids. Omega-3s are most commonly associated with fatty fish (salmon, trout, and tuna). But Omega-3s also can be found in soybean oil, grape seed (canola) oil, flaxseed oil, walnuts, Brussels sprouts, kale, spinach, and salad greens.

Trans Fats are one fat that should be *cut* entirely from your diet if possible. Since trans fats have been required to appear on food labels in the U.S., manufacturers have greatly reduced the amount of them in the food supply. Trans fats are almost entirely found in partially hydrogenated oils. These artificially hydrogenated oils have been found to have a strong negative impact on cardiovascular health. Foods containing less than 0.5g of trans fats per serving can have 0g of trans fat placed on the label. When purchasing baked goods and margarines, check the label to see if they contain any trans fats.

Bottom line Simple Changes:

- Choose fats from fish, vegetable oils (especially canola and olive), avocados and nuts most often.

- Choose fats from red meats, dairy (butter, cheese), in moderation.

- Avoid trans fats and be wary of products with low-fat, reduced-fat, and fat-free claims.

26. Walk Your Dog . . . First, Get A Dog

Ok, I admit that if you don't already have a dog this is not necessarily such a Simple Change. But so many studies point to having a dog as relieving stress, connecting you with something that loves you unconditionally, and even helping you become more fit. (17)

(A caveat here: owning or adopting a dog is a large undertaking. Consider and plan your lifestyle and also living space around having one before buying a pet or even better adopting one from a shelter. Pet ownership of any kind is an important commitment. Make sure that you and your family, if you have one, understand the gravity of owning a pet. If you are not sure, don't do it. It's not fair to the animal.)

Dogs are simply love machines, pouring out grace with every wag of their tails! Yes, they need to be trained, and yes, they get sick and vomit on your expensive rug occasionally. They also need to be walked (or run) giving you *both* needed exercise. And they also can flood your brain with feel-good chemicals when you are petting them or playing with them.

Dogs also have an uncanny ability to know when it is time for you to take a break (about the same time they need to go out). They will wake you in the morning to exercise, and sometimes gently lull you to sleep. Having a dog is one of the most vitality-raising things you can do for yourself. (1) Get one. (2) Play with it. (3) Walk it. Repeat (2) and (3) daily—and watch your vitality rise.

27. Be Wise—Not Trendy—in your Diet

You can find a new fad diet pop up almost every week (if in doubt peruse *The New York Times* Bestseller List "How-To and Miscellaneous" section on Sundays.). The diets tout the latest trend on how to lose weight and get the super-model body you've always dreamed of in mere days or weeks. While these diets claim promising results, they are often faulty.

Diets using fasting principles can slow your metabolism over time, resulting in your body's burning fewer calories and trying to conserve extra body fat while depleting itself of nutrients.

Diets eliminating one or more major food groups (i.e. Wheat Belly) may help you lose weight in the beginning by reducing your calorie intake. However, deleting a whole food group makes it more challenging to get the proper nutrition and to stick to your diet while you are traveling, eating at restaurants, or eating with company. This diet can also be hard to maintain in the long run. Eventually when you quit a fad diet—and history shows you will—it will be hard to keep off the pounds you lost, often creating a "rebound" effect.

If you are trying to lose weight but the pounds aren't melting off as quickly as you dreamed, it's OK. Society's weight expectations and flood of weight-loss ads create an image that fast weight loss is ideal. But you should only lose about a pound or two a week on a realistic eating plan that includes exercise along with healthy eating. Losing weight too fast will result in weight loss from bone, water, and muscle in addition to burning away fat.

Consult a Registered Dietitian to help you get started on a healthy eating plan to reach your weight-loss goals. Remember that diet is one part of the picture. Exercise and taking care of your mental health are an important part of overall vitality and reaching your weight loss goals. Try looking on www.acefitness.org for a personal trainer (The American Council on Exercise), and www.eatright.org (Academy of Nutrition and Dietetics) for a Registered Dietitian.

28. Practice More Recovery Tools

Recovery is such an important part of vitality it deserves even more tools.

Some additional techniques I use with my clients include:

- Incorporating a deep breathing or meditation routine nightly to help break the stress cycle and sleep more restfully.
- Identifying and scheduling time to unplug totally from your technology at least three times every week for at least two hours at a time in the beginning stages of your Simple Changes. Translation: "Unplugging totally" means leaving your smart phone at home. (If you can't completely unplug from, say, family, have a back-up phone used only for them.)
- Developing a ritual to physically and mentally end your workday and disengage from the workplace.

29. Train Your Brain

There is a reason for the huge increase in books and media around mindfulness, meditation and training your brain. Our brains are on overload, and there is little down time for them to replenish what they need and actually grow new neural connections. This Simple Change is a win/win. If you take even short periods of time to focus on both exercising your brain and providing it with true rest, you will find so many benefits. It's now widely recognized that through mental simulations and exercises there is huge potential for neuroplasticity—brain's ability to change itself. In case you are wondering, the changes seen in simulations did transfer over to real life, *if* they were done on a regular basis. There are a number of books and even apps and websites to guide you in training your brain. In Appendix 3 are some of those resources to help you along the way.

Among the benefits of training your brain (with practices like Yoga, meditation, brain training games, mindfulness practice, and focused breathing (to name a few) include:

- Improved memory recall
- Increased neural connections

- Greatly reduced risk of diseases like dementia, and Alzheimer's
- Increased brain size
- Better socialization skills
- The ability to relax upon demand
- Ability to focus in key situations for longer periods of time.

Enough studies have been done to date to prove that exercising your brain is equally—if not more important than exercising your body.

30. Focus

The need for focus is so critical particularly in a world where concentration—because of technology and information overload—becomes even more important and more difficult. Today's adults and children have been called by many experts the "ADD generation," partially as a result of too many stimuli. It does not have to be this way but only you can make the difference in yourself.

Improved focus, among many other things—improves our "presence" with people, helps us work more error free, quiets the internal chatter in our minds, and prevents the release of stress hormones and adrenaline associated with multi—tasking. One study found that office distractions eat an average of 2.1 hours per day for individuals in the workplace. (18) This study also showed that the average worker spent an average of only 11 minutes per day before being interrupted, and that it takes 20 minutes to fully engage on the task they were working on before the interruption, if they do at all!

You can control your focus or be controlled by distraction. It is your decision. Here are some of my clients' best tips:

- Schedule at least 45 minutes of uninterrupted think time each day.
- Do a breathing or meditation (free of technology) before going into a meeting or critical presentation.

- Set aside e-mail until you have completed at least one important task.
- Volunteer outside of work—give with your time, not just a check.
- Handwrite at least one personal note per week in gratitude.
- Schedule and accomplish "one big thing" each day.

31. Plan for Healthy Eating at Work

Once Monday morning gets started it is important to remember your commitment to eat healthfully.   Meetings run long; interruptions happen, and many other factors conspire against healthy eating. Know this and plan for it.   A hugely important tip I can give to you is this: *Never get too tired, hungry or thirsty without being prepared!* Some favorite client tricks include:

- Scheduling extra "food energy" breaks during meetings for your team.
- Providing a branded water bottle for prospects/client engagements and using them!
- Bringing extra healthy energy snacks to meetings and while traveling. Share them with clients and co-workers (notice their reaction!)
- Using on-site opportunities to take team members—or clients— to healthy restaurants. Plan ahead.
- Replacing the receptionist's candy jar with fresh fruit, or raw, unsalted almonds.
- Ordering-in healthy foods for snack/lunch breaks at meetings.

32. Use A "Go To" Cookbook

Just as there are many "diet" books (just check *The New York Times* bestseller list if you doubt it), there are several very healthy and easy (less-than-20-minute recipes) cookbooks available as well. Go online, or to your local bookstore and peruse the cooking section. Look for books that use natural ingredients and have recipes that are quick and easy to prepare (and look appetizing to you). Cooking from an easy and healthful cookbook will:

- Make cooking much simpler
- Provide you with complete macro nutrients
- Give you the satisfaction of doing something healthy for you and your family
- Save money on eating out.

Commit to cooking from one of these cookbooks at least twice a week to start with versus eating fast food or going out to a calorie-dense dinner. I've listed some resources of cookbooks my clients like in Appendix 3—resources I hope that will get you started.

33. Prepare Your Exercise Gear the Night Before

I know. This is one you've heard before, probably more than once. There is a reason: It works. How many times have you gone to bed with a promise to yourself that you'll wake up 45 minutes early and go for a run, walk, class, or _____(fill in the blank) the following morning? Or before you go to the office, saying that you'll do one of the above as soon as you get home? Then you may have often hit the snooze button, or turned on the TV, opened the mail, or begun doing something else distracting only to lose your motivation.

This is a pivotal moment in your attempt to gain some momentum with your exercise program. First of all, you are not alone. Many of us have the best intentions in mind until we wake up and it's still dark, or get home dead tired and make a few excuses that keep us from exercising.

Laying out your entire workout outfit, or packing your fitness bag and *putting it in a place where you can't help but notice it* can often motivate you to get going. In the morning, put your gear near your bed or in your bathroom. In the afternoon lay it out right inside your front door—essentially somewhere where you will actually stumble over it! Try this technique if you are having trouble getting started (even if you feel silly at first). It works.

34. Manage You Team's Recovery Time

If you are a leader it is critical that you build in times for recovery for your whole team when they are working on a project. There is a reason that companies like Google have pool and ping-pong tables in their common areas. All of us, particularly in these times of heavy work demands, need breaks that totally separate us from our work and foster more energy.

The benefits of team recovery time are similar to building in your own recovery time and provide a much-needed break for the brain.

If you are a manager/leader, ask your team what they would like to have in the way of breaks, then get any tools that may facilitate healthy breaks for them. They *will* tell you. In addition to taking care of your team, you will be viewed as a leader who keeps his or her team motivated without burning them out.

35. Invest in Exercise Equipment

Exercising at home is one of the biggest excuse killers that I know of. Fully 65 percent of my clients own home exercise equipment. Also, home exercise equipment has become much more affordable in the past decade. For instance where quality treadmills used to cost upwards of $1,500, you can now find a sturdy, fully programmable one for under $1,000. Generally speaking, if you are buying home equipment you'll want to start with a sturdy piece of cardiovascular equipment such as a treadmill, elliptical trainer, or bike.

Space and cost will factor into this equation as well as—and very importantly— your preferred form of exercise. If you don't like cycling, a stationary cycle will become a clothes dryer in very short order.

I always recommend starting with a quality piece of cardiovascular equipment and adding other equipment choices as budget allows. That's because cardiovascular exercise is one of the most important types, and the equipment is among the most costly. Other equipment for strength and flexibility can be much less costly and very space-efficient. Some very effective additional pieces include:

- Dumbbells or kettle bells
- Exercise mat
- DVD's (Yoga, flexibility, etc.)
- Heartrate monitor
- Strength building rubber tubing.

Working out at home requires no gym fees, travel times, and no one cares what you look like! Shop around and always, always, try the equipment before you buy it and compare warranties. Many equipment manufacturers have DVD's or YouTube videos available to help you get started. Additionally, you can use resources like The American Council on Exercise website, www.acefitness.org/acefit/fitness-programs/, for exercise ideas.

36. Be ADD No More!

We are often called a society of ADD individuals—so much so that many of us are pretty sick of this moniker. The science suggests that the amount of stimuli available to us on a constant basis might be the reason. (19) We have smart phones, tablets, laptops, and the

Internet that in many cases are always on. It's also been shown in some studies that humans are not equipped to multi-task and that doing so means we are not doing one thing at a time with the proper amount of focus. (20)

Focus in this new environment will not happen on its own. You must provide the space for it. Here are some suggestions to strengthen your focus muscles:

- Turn off your auto e-mail function. Designate certain times each day that you will check it.
- During long meetings ask for and take strategic breaks where you can walk for 10 minutes, get something healthy to snack on and give your brain a rest (the key here is getting up).
- Train yourself (a little bit at a time) to turn off all technology particularly at home so you can focus on what is happening around you in the present moment.
- Before an important phone call, presentation, or meeting, take 3 to 5 minutes to close your eyes, breathe deeply and count your breaths (count from 1 to 8, repeating again after each 8 count during those 3 to 5 minutes). Make sure all of your technology is on mute or standby for even a few minutes while doing this or even better try to change your surroundings.
- Use your commuting time to turn off your phone or tablet and focus on something enjoyable like pleasurable audio reading or music to ease into the evening.
- If you are holding a meeting, stick to the time limits that you set at the beginning. Generally speaking, meetings over an hour become something less than effective.
- Consider 5 minute stretch and water breaks to help you hold your focus and that of your team's.

Focus is hugely important to us for better work, relationships with others, and relationships with ourselves. Create space for yours.

37. Change Up Your Exercise

How often have you exercised for long periods of time doing the same routine only to find that your body is no longer responding? Almost always this is because you have hit a plateau that you cannot seem to break through whether your goal is weight management, strength, or flexibility—to name a few. Here's the deal: almost all experts agree that making gains in your fitness routine involves 2 things: 1) making periodic changes to the type of exercises you are doing, and 2) increasing the intensity of your exercise.

(A reminder: *intensity* means something different to every *body*. If you are an experienced exerciser it will perhaps mean running at a higher heart rate for part of your workout for instance. If you are older or a new exerciser it might be simply increasing the incline a degree or two on a treadmill. Bottom line is to use intensity sensibly.) I covered intensity in the first 5 Quick-Start changes, so here's more about making changes to your routine.

Let me give you an example: Say your goal is weight loss. You are used to walking on the treadmill at a steady pace for 30 minutes 4 times per week at a certain speed. You've been doing this for 6 months or longer and don't seem to be getting anywhere. Chances are that your body adjusted to the pace and time several months ago and is now conserving calories. Essentially, the body, in its infinite wisdom, has said, "oh this is how much were going to stretch our systems" and adapted by burning no more energy than is absolutely needed.

If this sounds like you, the challenge is to change things up. Start using an elliptical trainer, rower, or even adding one of the other programs on the treadmill into your routine. This should be done at least two out of the three days you are exercising. This same principal goes for strength training and flexibility. On at least one to three of your workout days try some new exercises or even a new mode of exercise, e.g. Yoga.

Generally speaking it's best to change things up at least every 6 to 8 weeks. Keep in mind that these changes do not have to be drastic but simply something different than what you've been doing.

38. Take Food Energy Breaks

Based on our circadian rhythms, our energy waxes and wanes in tune with our own specific rhythms. Learn to listen to yours and when you are on the downside of an energy "wave" take a snack break to minimize the effect. For your breaks, eat only foods that help stabilize your energy, like:

- Plain almonds
- Hummus and whole grain bread
- Peanut butter and whole grain bread sandwiches
- Trail mix
- Low sugar, high fiber, energy bars
- Whole fruits—not juices
- Greek yogurt topped with fresh fruit or granola
- Strawberries with peanut butter

39. Hit the Pause Button at Least Twice a Day

This change can be a difficult one given the pace of our daily lives and for that matter our culture. We are expected (or expect of ourselves) to get as much done as is humanly possible most days of the week. Whether it's a project at work, or tending to the needs of our families we can very easily become mired in endless tasks or "to do" lists. Running on this "treadmill" creates long-term physical and mental negative effects on our bodies and our minds, from depression to hypertension and worse.

We are designed to take breaks after a series of chores or tasks but many of us have forgotten that—sometimes long ago. What was once called recess is now considered wasted time. Indeed, it is not. Our brains and our bodies need breaks according to our natural rhythms—each being unique to each individual. These breaks of even10-15 minutes to call a friend, take a walk, or just sit out in a setting with natural light can bring enormous short and long term effects. These "pauses" help our brains process newly gained information, create new neural pathways, and in the end, make us smarter. They also lift our moods, and in cases where we do manual work certainly give our bodies a respite and help us to work more safely.

Getting in the habit of hitting the pause button is not easy. Everything around us suggests that we power through on a daily basis. As mentioned earlier however, the cost of doing so can be very high. Schedule pauses *at least* every 90 minutes and take them!

40. Vary Your Veggies

Studies have shown that when people are presented with a variety of foods they tend to serve larger portions and in turn eat more (21). This propensity has often been shown with candy. For example, with M&M's people will take larger portions when all colors are mixed together versus a bowl of all red M&M's. Why not make this tendency work in your favor to increase your vegetable intake? Instead of having just broccoli or green beans, have a vegetable melody. Get as many colors as you can try:

- Broccoli, carrots, cauliflower
- Zucchini, red peppers, mushrooms
- Asian stir-fry blend
- Italian medley

Even check the freezer section for vegetable mixes that are ready to be cooked in minutes.

41. Feel Your Fullness

To liberate yourself from unhealthy portion sizes, think about the last meal you ate. Why did you stop eating? For many people, the answer is "when the food was gone" or "when I cleaned my plate." With busy schedules, people often wait until they are starving to devour a meal in minutes—resulting in overeating and feeling bloated. It's easy to find yourself eating out of routine without acknowledging what's going on in your body.

I challenge you to focus on how you feel before you sit down to a meal and after you're done. Try to grab something to eat when you *just start* to feel hungry or have slight stomach rumblings but before you are famished or feeling light-headed. Pace yourself as you are eating. If you are eating during a lunch meeting, try putting your fork down in between bites and while talking. This change will help you to slow down your eating and allow you to start to feel full.

When you are done think about how you feel. Are you satisfied or do you feel bloated or stuffed? If you are feeling bloated or stuffed that's a signal from your body that you ate more than you needed for that meal. Next time you may need to slow down a little more to give your body time to feel full and to signal you to stop eating sooner.

If you aren't ready to focus on how you feel before, during, and after you eat try this instead. Stop when you still have 1/3 of your food left. At that point decide if you are still hungry or feeling full before you continue to eat.

Use the scale below to help you determine your "satiety level" and feel more in touch with your body's hunger and satiety cues. Begin eating when you are at a 2 on the scale of 1 - 5. Stop eating when you are approaching a 3. You should start to feel more comfortable and satisfied but not yet completely full. As your food digests you will typically feel more full 5 to 10 minutes after you finished eating than you did while you were eating. You won't have to use this scale forever, just until you think that you have mastered your hunger "feelings."

Hunger/Fullness Scale

1. **Starving**—Very uncomfortable. Feeling irritable and unable to concentrate; weak & light-headed.
2. **Slightly Hungry**—A little uncomfortable. Beginning to feel signs of hunger.
3. **Neutral**—Comfortable. More/less satisfied; could eat a little more but don't need to.
4. **Full**—A little bit uncomfortable.
5. **Bloated/nauseous**—Uncomfortably full. Need to loosen clothes.

42. Watch Your Plate

Being smart about *portion control* is another key Simple Change. It's estimated the average dinner plate has increased 36% in size over the last 50 years both in the home and at restaurants (22). It's no wonder obesity rates have been skyrocketing at a record pace during that period of time (23). We often feel we need to, or should, eat what is served to us or what we put on our plates. One cup of rice will leave more space on a 12 inch plate than an 8 inch plate. This empty space cues us that there is more room, and most people will end up serving themselves a larger portion.

Take a look at the plate you eat from at home, chances are it's around 12 inches in diameter, while you may have "salad" plates around that are 8 inches or 9 inches in diameter. Switch it up and start eating your meals from the 8 to 9 inch plate. On average, people will serve themselves 22% less food on a smaller plate (24). Whether we are serving ourselves on a small or large plate, we tend to eat about 90% of what we serve ourselves (25).

If you don't have smaller plates and aren't looking to buy new ones, try using disposable 8 or 9 inch plates for a week. See if you find yourself eating less at meals as a result. If you are unsure think about how you feel after the meal. Do you typically feel 'bloated' or 'stuffed' and now find yourself just comfortably full or satisfied instead?

The benefits are many when you have mastered this including:

- Much better control at home and especially in restaurants in knowing when you are full
- Much easier weight management or weight loss
- Less of a chance of filling up with empty calories (usually carbohydrates)
- Having a feeling of satiety vs. feeling heavy or sluggish after eating
- Improved energy and fewer highs and lows throughout the day
- Improved sleep (no more heavy dinners!).

43. Go for an Upper-Body Run or Walk

Running and walking are two of the best forms of exercise. They have great cardiovascular benefit, and because they are weight bearing (as opposed to say cycling, or rowing) they have some benefit for strengthening the muscles and bones in the lower body. Additionally most of us can accomplish one or the other. Unfortunately, they do little of the same for the upper body.

Buy a 4 foot rubber tube with handles on each end (found at any sporting goods store), tie it around your waist, and go out for your walk or run. At different points during the walk, stop and complete some shoulder presses, biceps, or triceps exercises, or any other upper body strength exercise that you can think of. For ideas go to the American Council on Fitness website, www.acefitness.org/acefit/fitness-programs/, for some additional strength training ideas. Remember that strength training thickens bone density, and creates caloric burning lean muscle mass.

44. Engage A Personal Trainer . . . For Free!

Now that I have your attention here is how it works. Think about your friends and acquaintances—the ones that either currently work out or want to. Before you contact anyone, identify the ones who seem to always follow through on their promises. This follow-through is crucial. If you choose someone who is not usually accountable, you run the risk of him or her not working out—literally. Let the person you choose know that you are committed to starting a vitality program and ask if he or she would be interested in doing so with you. Have a formal meeting where you discuss each other's goals and available times. *Also* discuss any limitations that either of you have such as time, space, injury, or other barriers to success.

Determine if you can be each other's partner for exercising, controlling stress, even eating. Discuss what that "partnering" may look like and decide if there is a fit. If there is, look at each other's schedules for at least a month in advance. (Going forward, do this each and every month.). Determine what exercise classes you might want to attend, cooking classes, etc. *Put them in your calendar and treat them as you would any other appointment.*

From time to time, "true up" with each other. Has one or the other been less accountable? If so why, and can that be changed? An honest dialogue must be had in order for this Simple Change to work. *So much of living vitally is about showing up* and it can help so much having a partner; if it works out you'll each have your own personal trainer!

45. Stick To Your Schedule

Having a plan that makes your life work includes trying to keep your mind and body in a state that allows for consistency and balance. This means being consistent in all things vital including your sleep, times that you eat, exercise, and work. Try to stick your schedule for all of the above except when you travel for vacation and work. This regularity will help you stay refreshed, alert, and add immeasurably to your vitality. If you do have to deviate from this regular schedule try to get back to it as soon as you can, e.g. post travel and other irregularities that life throws your way.

Smartphones and other technology can help greatly with regular schedules by helping you to set alarms for everything from snacking to acting as an alarm clock in the morning.

46. Just Move!

Recent studies link heart disease, diabetes and other lifestyle-related disorders to sitting for more than two hours at a time!(26) Unless you walk and stand for a living try some of the following tips. Get up from sitting at least every two hours and walk—even if it's just around your house or office. Try to set up a workstation with computer that allows you to stand while working. If you want to take this further, now you can even buy treadmills that are equipped with desks so you can walk while working.

Humans are not designed to sit for long periods of time, and yet for many of us everything we do conspires to have us do so. Try to find ways in your life that accommodate standing and moving more.

47. Use Caffeine Wisely

Caffeine can help us improve our concentration, hold it longer and also keep us more alert when we need it. Consuming as little as 37.5 mg of caffeine (half a cup of coffee) has been reported to improve alertness, short-term recall and reaction time, positive reported mood and lower perceived fatigue. (27) Experts vary as to the proper amounts daily. However, a moderate daily intake of less than 250 mg of caffeine is considered safe to consume habitually. (28) In general, an upper limit of 400 mg per day is set to lower the risk of more serious health effects. But side effects can be seen with over 250 mg of caffeine. Too much caffeine can trigger headaches, irritability, anxiety and a host of other biological and psychological problems including heart problems. People who are sensitive to caffeine may notice these negative effects with lower doses.

Experiment with the amount of caffeine you consume daily and perhaps even keep a journal for a few days to determine how much is right for you to perform your daily activities from exercise to working. If our client's journals are correct, we generally consume more than we actually *think* we do. Keeping a journal will help keep your intake honest.

And, oh, 24 ounce lattes with other additives are not a healthy way to get our caffeine. Some of these drinks add to weight gain and over caffeinating. Some of them also give us as much as more than two-thirds of the recommended daily total caloric intake for a whole day in one drink! Stick to no more than two 8 ounce cups a day with little or no cream or sugar. Also, be wise when ordering and using caffeine and read labels to look for hidden sources of caffeine, particularly later in the day as this can affect your sleep.

Most experts, including the National Sleep Foundation, recommend not having caffeinated beverages or foods after 2:00 p.m. daily. (29)

Caffeine Content of Beverages

Beverage	Size (fl oz)	Caffeine (mg)
Espresso	1	64
Coffee, brewed	8	95
Coffee, instant	8	62
Black Tea	8	47
Green Tea	8	44
Cola	12	33
5-Hour Energy	2	207
Red Bull	8.4	77

Data retrieved from USDA National Nutrient Database for Standard Reference

Release 27, http://ndb.nal.usda.gov/.

48. Exercise Your Core

You've probably read and heard a lot about core exercise as of late. Core exercise relates to strengthening your stomach, hip, buttocks, and low back muscles in a way that will keep you from injury and even help you stand erect. Aside from all that has been written, it's really quite simple. Go online and look at some YouTube core exercise routines to get a sense of how they work and how you can incorporate them into your day. Another even better idea is to hire a Certified Personal Trainer for at least 3 sessions to assess your posture and muscle weaknesses and help you with a program for your personal core muscles. Another is to join a Yoga class—a discipline that really concentrates on your core—with a certified Yoga instructor.

Humans weren't meant to walk around with our heads and necks forward and our shoulders hunched but often do as a result of reading, keyboard, texting, and other modern-day activities. Slouching this way has been linked to everything from joint stiffness, arthritis, muscle aches, and even difficulty breathing. And standing tall and walking erect sends a message of vitality to the rest of the world. Core training can help this immeasurably.

Making exercises for your core a habit at least three times per week is a truly worthwhile use of your time. These can be done in as little as 5 to 10 minutes per session and require no equipment. In Appendix 5 I have included safe and effective examples to start with. These exercises can be done in any setting and don't require exercise clothing so that they can be done with limited time even in a hotel or office setting or perhaps even while watching the news or a favorite show on TV. I've also provided some apps that use these and other core exercises in Appendix 3. Stand tall!

49. Use Apps For Health and Vitality

As I write I have 36 apps on my smart phone that help me do everything from Yoga while traveling to sitting and breathing properly (while clearing my mind). There are apps that will track your eating and fitness. There are apps that will take you through a core workout, and others take you through a full workout regime. There are apps that will help you chart your progress over time, which can be immensely helpful. Finding apps that are right for you will definitely take some time (and trial and error). I recommend first defining your goals. (See the Reaching Your Vitality Goals Exercise in Appendix 1). I promise you that the time you spend in customizing your phone for the right ones will return your time many-fold.

As you browse sample some, and in some cases let your intuition guide you. In Appendix 3 I have also provided the names of some apps that my clients have found most useful.

50. Get Stronger in Small Bits

Remember that you do not have to do all of your strength training (for the whole body) in one session. Find small pockets of time during the morning, day, or evening where you can do even 1 to 2 sets of an exercise so that by bedtime you have covered most of your major muscle groups, including chest, back, shoulders, triceps, biceps, abdominals, and legs.

As with other Simple Changes, it will help greatly to have your resistance tubing or dumbbells handy when you have a moment, although body weight exercises count as well. Both tubing and dumbbells are very inexpensive, so consider having a few sets around in places where you'll likely use them during convenient times. Some of our client's favorite locations include:
- Near the TV
- In the kitchen
- In the office
- In the family room
- In a briefcase or carryon (for the bands).

51. Get Out of the Hotel

One of the greatest pleasures of travel is walking or jogging around a city. You'll be getting your dose of exercise and will see things that normal tourists never do. It's helpful to keep an energy bar and some money with your gear in case you get hungry or lost. Google Maps is an absolute wonder for helping you navigate a foreign (or foreign to you) city. But I must tell you that sometimes getting lost is half the fun! Try to exercise as soon as you arrive at your destination (if it is during the day). This activity will help give you some Vitamin D, and also help you adjust to the time zone. If you prefer exercising indoors inquire before the trip about the exercise facility *including* the times that it is open for use.

Just like laying your exercise clothes out in advance of a scheduled session, preparing for exercising on the road is crucial. Keep a dedicated exercise outfit in your carryon suitcase *all the time*. Keep it simple: a t-shirt, shorts, or tights, socks and walking or running shoes. Before you leave check the weather and add layers, gloves, hats, accordingly if you are an outdoor exerciser.

52. Do Something To Give Back

Think about your favorite charity. Now go to their website or contact them about upcoming events. Likely there is a fun 5k walk or run or something else that counts as helping them out while increasing your vitality. Even delivering meals to the elderly or taking someone with dementia for a walk can be a great ways to exercise your vitality while helping someone with theirs. If you don't see activities like these or others available come up with one yourself. Doing so will be great for your body and your mind. If you've done this before you'll know that it provides needed recovery and will even help your body release hormones that are associated with a better mood and disposition.

On a larger scale, giving back can provide a deeper sense of meaning to your life, and also the feeling of love that comes from giving to others who are in need. It is important to choose something that you truly are committed to. I love this quote from Steven Covey, the author of *The 7 Habits of Highly Effective People*: "Don't show me where you spend your money. Show me where you spend your time." In other words, jump into a project with your favorite charity—mentally and physically. Donate your time and vitality not just your money.

53. Find A Trusted Physician

Health care these days (as if I had to tell you!) is very tricky indeed. It is so important to be able to speak with your doctor candidly, have the ability to communicate when you are not there, be able to get trusted referrals from him/her when necessary and get *all* of your questions and worries addressed on an ongoing basis.

As I said, this can be tricky. There are many M.D.s out there who are outstanding, but who are simply overwhelmed with patients and short on time. Choose wisely. Ask questions like: How can I reach you or communicate when we don't have an appointment? Keep a medical log on your computer that includes dates of visits, critical information, and questions that you will want to ask on your next visit. Many physicians use e-mail now, so you can even ask questions without an appointment. In these cases make sure that your questions are very specific, including providing examples of symptoms where applicable.

In short, it is absolutely critical that you are proactive in your relationship with your doctor. If you aren't who will be?

54. Be Open to Alternative Health Care—With Care

The science now shows us clearly that alternative healing works. Organizations like The Clinical Psychology Division of The American Psychology Association now support the benefits of certain alternative healing practices. (30) There are also numerous studies that show that acupuncture, chiropractic care, massage and a host of other disciplines can be very helpful for everything from Fibromyalgia, to back pain, even migraines. (31) Most of alternative care is non-invasive and can take up where Western medicine leaves off. However, choosing the right practitioner is *absolutely essential* and the best place to start (often) is with your primary care physician. Many of my clients have used alternative healers who were recommended by their M.D.'s with great success, and western medicine is becoming much more proactive about this type of care. The next best place to find referrals is through friends or acquaintances, preferably those who have similar issues as yours.

A few other things to consider:
- Is the healer certified/licensed by a national or global entity?
- Has he or she worked with patients with your ailment before?
- Can he or she provide you with patients' names and phone numbers as references?
- Is the facility clean and orderly?

Alternative healing is essentially become less "alternative" and more "primary" than ever before. There's a reason.

55. Add Yoga or Pilates

I have found that good basic exercise principals that are "fad free" are always the best in the long run. I also feel very strongly that Yoga and Pilates are excellent adjuncts for any adult looking to having better posture, a healthier spine, more mobile joints, and better balance (to name just a few). I regularly recommend adding Yoga or Pilates at least 2 days per week.

There are essentially two ways you can start one of these practices: The first—and generally the best, at least to begin with—is to seek out a studio or gym that has instructors certified in one of the disciplines you are seeking to explore. Then take at least two classes (often complimentary) before committing more time and dollars. Things to look for if you are exploring a class:

- Is the instructor certified by a nationally accredited association?
- Does the instructor provide clear instructions and also properly demonstrate and correct the movements?
- Does the instructor provide individual attention to participants in making sure that a posture or movement is done correctly?
- Does the instructor show alternative postures or movements for those with limited mobility or other restrictions?

Another way to access these disciplines is through DVDs and apps. It's important to be very careful when choosing one of these mediums. Do some research on who has created the app or DVD: Is he or she a certified instructor? Are the instructions clear? Does the instructor show alternative postures or movements?

Some of my clients' self-reported benefits from Yoga and Pilates that they have shared with me include:

- Increased relaxation and better sleep
- Better focus and concentration
- Much greater flexibility
- Better digestion
- The ability to be more "in the moment"
- Better balance for daily activities and sports.

These exercise disciplines are very worthwhile, especially as we age.

56. Find Your Inner Athlete

Every one of us has an inner athlete just waiting to be recognized. Even if you were not athletic when you were young, or think you are too old (you are not!), you are an athlete —like all of your ancestors. Maybe you just need to find your sport for whatever stage of life you find yourself. These days you can find places to golf, bowl, water-ski, play Ultimate Frisbee, and even join fun runs that include your dog!

Participating in a sport has so many benefits beyond the physical realm. It can help to distract you from work or problems, provide much needed light and fresh air, and improve your self-esteem immeasurably. Now I'm not expecting you to strap on pads and go out for an adult football team (although those exist). I'm encouraging you to try a sport that you are drawn to. You do not have to win, you simply must show up. So find your athlete!

57. Conquer Buffets

Buffets can be a challenging battleground if you are trying to eat well, especially while watching your waistline. The endless supply of variety can lead even the most conscious person to unwittingly overindulge.

If you know you'll be eating at a buffet later in the day, stick to your regular eating routine throughout the day. If you go to the buffet famished you are more likely to overeat than if you are simply moderately hungry. Try to get a table farthest from the buffet and sit with your back to the food. If you are not looking at the food you may have passed up the first time, you are more likely to forget about it and suppress the urge to go for a second helping. Before you grab your plate, take a minute to just walk around the buffet. Choose the items that you'll enjoy the most and don't have a chance to eat on a regular basis.

Don't forget to pick vegetables. Just because you are at a buffet doesn't mean you can't eat well. Start with a salad with lots of color. Mix up lettuce, carrots, broccoli, radishes and more. Take it easy on the cheese, croutons, bacon bits, and dressing that can easily turn your light salad into a full meal.

Plate it smart. Make half of your main plate vegetables, one-fourth of your plate protein, and one-fourth starch (like pasta salad, rice pilaf, mashed potatoes—preferably whole grains), following the suggestions on www.choosemyplate.gov.) When in doubt stay away from white starches.

If you are going to go back for seconds keep your first plate on the table as a visual reminder of what you already ate. If you have a sweet tooth, plan for your dessert by eating less starchy foods you normally would during the main course and stop before you are full. Pick out your favorite treat that you know you'll be able to savor and enjoy. If you can't make up your mind, try splitting a couple of treats with someone else.

Also remember to eat slowly and enjoy those around you. Drink water before your meal and sip during. To prevent yourself from mindlessly eating, set your fork down in between bites and while talking to your company.

58. Snack Smart

Often clients will try to not eat between meals when trying to eat well. But if you are going long hours between meals (generally more than five hours) or are active throughout the day, snacking can be beneficial. Waiting too long between meals can cause you to over-eat later in the day or even during the night. Potentially even more damaging, going too long without eating can leave you feeling tired, groggy, and maybe a little grumpy due to your stomach's rumbling and having low blood sugar.

Follow these tips for snacking when you have five or more hours between meals: Have a snack that combines carbohydrates (sugar, starch, bread) and protein (eggs, nuts, meats). Carbohydrates are the preferred source of energy for your brain. Having carbohydrates will help keep you thinking sharp and feeling awake. However, having only or mostly carbohydrates (especially sugars, and other "white starches") can leave you feeling even hungrier, causing you to overeat. Add protein to snacks in order to feel full and maintain muscle mass.

Try these ideas for snacks under 250 calories:

- 1 pc wheat bread + 1 tablespoon peanut butter
- 1 apple + 1 Baby Bell cheese round
- 1 banana + 12 almonds
- ¼ cup (1 small box) raisins + 1/8 cup peanuts
- 8 dried apricot halves + 10 walnut halves
- 1 6-oz yogurt cup
- 10 baby carrots + 10 Wheat Thins + 2 tablespoons hummus.

If you are looking for other snack ideas or checking the labels on your snack bars look for about 15 grams of carbohydrate and *at least* 7 grams of protein for a small snack.

59. Order Healthy In-Flight Food

Traveling can wreak havoc on your entire system. Not only are you likely to be lacking sleep and rest but also it can be challenging to find healthy food choices. Airline food has come a long way in recent years by marketing healthier choices to fliers. Many airlines have complete fresh-style meals available in flight. Look for some of the options below on your next flight (or purchase them in the airport before you board).

For breakfast choose:
- Whole fresh fruit with Greek yogurt
- Eggs, whole wheat toast, fruit.

For lunch or dinner choose:
- Whole meats (chicken breast, steak) instead of cured processed meats like deli ham or charcuterie meats
- A meal with a side of fruit or vegetables for a source of fiber, vitamins and minerals.

If you are on a short flight and/or have a short connection you may not have time to grab a meal in the airport, and airline pickings maybe slim. Plan ahead with some snack ideas to bring from home. Select:

- Trail mix
- Whole or dried fruit
- Freeze-dried vegetables
- Nuts (pre-portioned into snack-size bags)
- Nut butters (travel packs)
- Whole-grain pretzels or crackers
- Snack bars (7g Protein, or pair a low-calorie bar with nuts).

Keep an eye out for the following airport snacks that can often be found close to terminals in easy-to-transport containers:

- Part-skim mozzarella cheese sticks
- Sandwich with lean meat, vegetables and mustard on whole-grain bread
- Salad with lean protein
- Fruit cup
- Pre-cut veggies (paired with nut butter from home)
- Hummus and whole-grain pita chips
- Yogurt.

60. Stay Smart with Fast Food

Even when on the road with time for only short stops, there are smart options to be found. In fast-food chains and convenience stores, choose from these smarter options:

- Pre-cut vegetables
- Hummus
- Yogurt (Greek style is a good choice)
- Sandwiches with whole grain breads

- Salads with lean meats and a variety of vegetables—or topped with seasonal fruits and nuts
- Fruit with peels, such as oranges and bananas.

If you are really craving a fast food favorite such as fries or a milkshake, choose the small or "kid's size" and savor your treat. Plus you'll save money!

Also, most fast food chains have calorie counts posted on the menu board or available behind the counter, so check out the calorie count. When in doubt look for items that are grilled, steamed, broiled or baked instead of fried or sautéed.

61. Conquer Jet Lag

Traveling is often accompanied by long nights and long hours that can take a toll on your body. Give extra attention to eating healthy and staying hydrated a few days before you travel to keep your body in top shape.

Heavy travelers need to be particularly aware of finding enough sleep, which may include naps wherever possible. Travel, next to having a newborn baby, provides the biggest challenge to your sleep. Generally speaking, crossing two or more time zones can wreak havoc with your sleep patterns.

Your body's internal clock, or circadian rhythm, does not like to change. So a time-change can leave you feeling groggy, even if you get your normal number of hours of sleep. For example, even if you got 8 hours of sleep, you will undoubtedly feel the effects if you are waking up at 4 am your local time (instead of your usual 7am). To lessen the shock to your body's natural rhythm try preparing for your trip before leaving. Two to three days before take-off try shifting your meal times an hour closer to the meal times of your destination. This will help your metabolism to adjust when you land at your destination, giving you a head start on beating jet lag. While at your destination adjust your meal times appropriately to keep your body in sync with the time zone change. These changes can give your body more time to adapt and decrease the effects of jet lag.

62. Eat Breakfast

Many people skip breakfast when they're in a rush or just because they simple don't feel hungry. But after a night's rest your body is in a "fasting" mode and needs to be fueled again to help jump-start your metabolism for the day. Eating breakfast can help reduce irritability and tiredness by providing your body with energy to use. A healthy breakfast can also help improve brain function, attention span, concentration, and memory. Start the morning off right with a breakfast that'll keep you energized and focused throughout the morning. Eating well in the morning can also help get you over those low energy humps more easily throughout the day.

Make breakfast simple by planning the night before and having foods ready to take in the car if necessary.

If you are not in the habit of eating breakfast you may not feel hungry in the morning so start with something small like a 6 oz. yogurt cup, a piece of fresh fruit, or a glass of 1% milk. It is important to have both carbohydrates and protein in your breakfast. Once you are in the habit of eating something in the morning you can start to make your breakfast more complete. Try:

- Oatmeal made with 1% milk with 1/2 frozen berries and 1 spoonful of sliced almonds
- Breakfast smoothie (1 cup 1% milk, ½ cup frozen fruit, 2 tablespoons nut butter)
- 2 hard-boiled eggs, 1 banana
- Peanut butter and banana sandwich with whole-grain bread

_ English muffin with 1 slice low-fat cheese and 2 slices of deli ham with a piece of fruit
_ Eggs with whole-grain toast and fruit.

In a rush–scramble two eggs with a splash of milk in a microwave safe container. Microwave for 30 seconds, stir and microwave again for 20 to 30 seconds, or make hard boiled eggs on your day off and store in the fridge for up to a week.

63. Have Your Sugar and Eat it Too!?

Most of us have at least a bit of a sweet tooth from time to time (sometimes often!). But we are all also familiar with the potentially hazardous effects of too much sugar: weight gain, increased risk of diabetes, poor lipid profile, etc. The World Health Organization currently recommends getting less than 5% of your calories from added sugars—about 25 grams of sugar per day. The average American gets about 90 grams of sugar (22.2 teaspoons) per day. (32)

"Added" sugar refers to sugars from sweeteners like corn syrup, sucrose, glucose, and maltose. But "added" does not include sugars that are found naturally in fruit and milk or in smaller quantities in grains. Determining how much sugar is *added* sugar, and how much is natural sugar on a label can be challenging. Skim labels for words ending in "—ose" or containing "syrup" to signal added sugars.

Feed your sweet tooth by choosing foods your will really enjoy and learn to savor them slowly. Watch your portion size and try these tips and dessert suggestions below.

If you are making sweets at home try to:
• Reduce the amount of sugar in baked goods by one- fourth
• Replace frosting with pureed fruit, fresh sliced fruit or a dusting of powdered sugar
• Use spices like nutmeg, cinnamon, or cardamom to add sweetness and flavor while using less sugar

Other ideas for eating less sugar:
- 2 Ghirardelli Chocolate squares + 10 walnut halves
- 1 Brownie (2x2 square) + 1 cup low fat milk
- Halved baked peaches with a sprinkle of brown sugar and cinnamon
- Split dessert at restaurants with 2 or more people
- Look for reduced sugar or fruit based dessert options.

64. Skip the OJ and Go Whole

Orange juice and other fruit juices may be an appealing way to get your daily fruit servings but may not be the wisest choice.

Particularly if you are diabetic or insulin resistant, fruit juice will cause a spike in blood sugar more pronounced than eating the whole fruit. One reason for the spike is that you will probably drink the juice faster than you would eat the whole fruit making you hungry sooner. Secondly, with the fruit broken down and the pulp usually removed the food is more rapidly digested. You are also more likely to consume more calories (and therefore more sugar) when drinking juice over eating the whole fruit. While a serving of fruit juice is one-half of a cup, most people will consume one cup or more. One cup of orange juice (240g) is 111 calories and 26 grams of carbohydrates while one large orange (184g) is 86 calories and 22 grams of sugar.

Since the orange will take longer to eat and typically will contain more fiber, it will help you to feel more full longer. To get the most out of your food and leave you feeling more satisfied choose whole fruits as often as possible.

65. Eat to Age Well

We all know that one person who looks about 10 years our junior, even though we're the same age. Usually it's attributed to good genes, but what if there's more to the story? What if you can act to protect your genes and slow aging? I'm not promising a one-shot fix or a miracle wrinkle reducer, but simply to help you slow the aging process.

Many studies and experts in nutrition have suggested that some foods may play a role in slowing the aging process. (33)While the research on aging is still young, it appears that nutritionists are zeroing in on some foods that can help. Foods that can help slow aging do so by protecting your cells from damage that occurs due to everyday processes. Foods that are high in anti-oxidants, omega-3 fatty acids, folate, and vitamin D may protect your current cells and help in the formation of new cells.

Anti-oxidants include:

- Vitamin C: citrus fruits (oranges, limes), tomatoes, potatoes, strawberries, leafy greens (spinach, arugula)
- Vitamin E: nuts (almonds, walnuts), seeds (pumpkin, flax), vegetable oils (canola, olive)
- Selenium: Brazil nuts, seafood, beef, dairy, rice and other grains

Other beneficial nutrients that may play a role include:

- Omega-3 fatty acids: flax seeds, walnuts, fatty fish (salmon, sardines)
- Folate: dark greens (spinach, asparagus, broccoli), lentils and beans (pinto, black, navy), fortified cereals and grains (enriched rice, breads, ready-to-eat cereals)
- Vitamin D: fatty fish (salmon, tuna, mackerel), dairy (milk), egg yolks, mushrooms

66. Eat for Working Out

To get the most out of your work-out you need to fuel both before and after. Eating right before will make sure you have plenty of energy to get you through your workout. Eating right after will help speed your recovery time and maximize muscle growth. Before your workout you want to have glucose (sugar) readily available to your body. If your last meal was less than three hours before exercise, you should be good to go for a moderate workout. If your last meal was more than three hours before, you may benefit from an extra snack to fuel your workout. Choose something light with 15-30g of carbohydrate. Try:

- 1 large banana
- 1 cup 1% milk
- ½ Peanut butter and jelly sandwich.

After your workout you need both carbohydrate and protein. Carbohydrate will be used to replenish your muscles stores of glycogen, the sugar used to fuel muscles. Protein is used to rebuild muscles. Especially when you've had a fairly hard strength training workout, you should get at least 20 grams of protein within an hour after. This 20 grams of protein is about 3 ounces of meat, poultry or fish, or 3 egg whites. If you are eating dinner in the next hour you'll likely get at least 20 grams of protein in your meal. However if it's going to be longer than an hour try one of these to snacks to hold you over:

- Cliff Bar Builders
- Protein shake, with a piece of fruit if the shake has less than 10 grams of carbohydrate
- 1 peanut butter and jelly sandwich + 1 cup milk
- 1 Greek yogurt cup + 2 tablespoons chopped nuts.

67. Shop Smart

Eating well at home starts at the grocery store. Plan your list *before* going to the store. And, more importantly, take your list with you and cross off items as you go. Decide to only buy what is on your list before going to the store to help reduce the risk of impulse buys for unnecessary items.

Do not go to the store hungry. Those chips will look much more appealing when you are thinking of a snack to eat on the way home than if you are already satisfied while shopping.

68. Add Needed Supplements

Over 50% of US adults take a nutritional supplement (34). Is a supplement right for you? Here are some guidelines:

- Vitamin D: Adults who do not get daily sun exposure or have dark skin may benefit from a Vitamin D supplement.
- Calcium: If you generally get less than 2 to 3 servings of dairy (1 cup milk, 1 ounce cheese) per day, then a calcium supplement may be right for you.
- B 12: If you are a vegan or over the age of 65 talk to your doctor about a B12 supplement.
- Omega 3/Fish oil: In many cases the benefits of an Omega 3 supplement are still unclear. Your best bet is to increase your intake of Omega 3s found in foods (walnuts, flax, and fish).
- I highly recommend consulting with a Registered Dietitian to help you create a personal eating plan for you.

69. Rearrange Your Dietary Environment

Foods that are in plain sight and easily accessible are more likely to be consumed (as if you didn't already know this!). Start placing treats like cookies, candies, and chips out of sight. Have space for them to be stored in the pantry or cupboard. Take out a serving of treats to eat and return the package to the cupboard *before* you enjoy your treat. I understand that this sounds obvious, but many, many clients have found that this Simple Change can make a large, long-term difference.

Take the opposite approach with fruit and vegetable snacks. Pre-wash and slice carrots, celery, and bell peppers for healthy snacks. Store them at eye level in your fridge in clear plastic containers. This will help them stand out when you are looking for something to munch on. Also keep a bowl of fresh fruit—also pre-washed—on your counter or work-space. Bottom line: make them easy to access and prepare.

70. Schedule a Standing Meal With a Friend

Huge vitality dividends can result from taking time and creating space around work and other responsibilities to simply engage in conversation and spending time with a friend on a *regular* basis. You take time away from your workspace or chores at home, while completely shifting the conversations (in your head and in real time) about what needs to be done or what you are *supposed* to be doing.

Also—trust me on this one—having a very objective listener who is not engaged in your work or other commitments can often open the door to new ways to solve those issues—sometimes without having the subjects even come up in conversation! This Simple Change is one of the most critical components of total vitality and one of the first to fall off of your calendar.

Make standing appointments with friends, and keep them. Watch what happens ....

Conclusion

Each person deserves to be vital—whatever that may look and feel like for you. For some it may be more energy; for others, to weigh less and move with more ease. I have provided some Simple Changes that, as they become habit will help you reach your personal goals.

Things will happen in your life—from impossible work deadlines to caring for a sick family member. These events sometimes have the effect of throwing you off your path to vitality. Worry not! These are called Simple Changes for a reason. Whenever you are ready, they are right here—waiting to be started again. And remember, it only takes 21 days for any of them to become a habit!

My wish for you is a long, healthy, and vital life.

Blessings,
Gregory Florez

Appendix 1

Reaching Your Vitality Goals Worksheet

Reaching Your Vitality Goals

Step One: State your vitality goal and intention, specifically and completely.

My Big Vitality Goal: _____

Specific Goals: List the top three things you want related to your goal above. What are some positive benefits to meeting your goal?

    1. _____

    2. _____

    3. _____

Step Two: Why? List up to 3 benefits this will bring to you personally- what will it allow you to do?

    1. _____

    2. _____

    3. _____

Step Three: Why haven't you reached your main Vitality goal? Complete the following statements with the first thing that comes to mind to help identify your barriers to success. What has kept you from reaching this goal?

The real reason I haven't is because: _____

I would take the necessary steps if only: _____

It is difficult for me because: _____

The one thing holding me back is: _____

If only I were: _____

It would help if: _____

Step Four: How? Brainstorm up to 3 possible *Simple Changes* you can make starting today.

1. _____
2. _____
3. _____

Step Five: Get Ready. List some tangible next steps you can commit to now.

1. _____
2. _____
3. _____

Step Six: Take Action! Act on one of these next steps each day/week.

Step Seven: How will you recognize your progress? _____

_____

_____

Appendix 2

Simple Changes for Specific Goals

Goal: Tuning Your Physical Self
- (3) 10 Minutes of Exercise Counts
- (6) Get Off "Automatic Pilot"
- (7) Make Your Exercise Intense
- (14) Take at least Three Walking Meetings per Week
- (16) Work with a Personal Trainer
- (21) Make Fitness a Priority
- (22) Get Inexpensive Exercise Equipment for Travel
- (26) Walk Your Dog . . . First Get a Dog
- (33) Prepare Your Exercise Gear the Night Before
- (35) Invest In Exercise Equipment
- (37) Change Up Your Exercise
- (43) Go for an Upper Body Run or Walk
- (44) Engage A Personal Trainer...For Free!
- (45) Stick to Your Schedule
- (46) Just Move!
- (48) Exercise Your Core
- (49) Use Apps for Health and Vitality
- (50) Get Stronger in Small Bits
- (51) Get Out of the Hotel
- (53) Find a Trusted Physician

(54) Be Open to Alternative Health Care—With Care

(55) Add Yoga or Pilates

(56) Find Your Inner Athlete

Goal: Eat Right. Live Light.

(1) Hydrate!

(2) Have Water and Healthy Food at Hand

(6) Get Off "Automatic Pilot"

(8) Prepare Your Eating Plan before the Week Begins

(12) Keep a Food Journal—A Short One

(23) Eat Fruits or Vegetables before Eating Out

(24) Alternate Water with Alcoholic Beverages

(25) Eat the Good Fats

(27) Be Wise—Not Trendy—in Your Diet

(31) Plan For Eating Healthy at Work

(32) Use a "Go To" Cookbook

(38) Take Food Energy Breaks

(40) Vary Your Veggies

(41) Feel Your Fullness

(42) Watch Your Plate

(47) Use Caffeine Wisely

(49) Use Apps for Health and Vitality

(57) Conquer Buffets

(58) Snack Smart

(59) Order Healthy In-Flight Food

(60) Stay Smart with Fast Food

(62) Eat Breakfast

(63) Have Your Sugar and Eat It Too!?

(64) Skip the OJ and Go Whole

(65) Eat To Age Well

(66) Eat for Working Out

(67) Shop Smart

(68) Add Needed Supplements

(69) Rearrange Your Dietary Environment

Goal: Recovery at Work and Home

(1) 10 Minutes of Exercise Counts

(2) Learn to Breathe Deeply

(3) Meditate for even 5 Minutes a Day

(6) Get Off "Automatic Pilot"

(9) Have a Recovery for Every Stressor

(10) Build in Recovery Time from Work to Home

(11) Develop a Bedtime Ritual

(14) Take at least three Walking Meetings per Week

(18) Do Your Work in Chunks

(19) Have Fun—Even a Little

(28) Practice More Recovery Tools

(34) Manage Your Team's Recovery Time

(36) Be ADD No More!

(38) Take Food Energy Breaks

(39) Hit the Pause Button At Least Twice a Day

(49) Use Apps for Health and Vitality

(52) Do Something to Give Back

(55) Add Yoga or Pilates

(61) Conquer Jet Lag

(70) Schedule a Standing Meal with a Friend

Goal: Creating a Vital, Mindful Brain

(1) Hydrate!

(4) Learn to Breathe Deeply

(5) Meditate for even 5 Minutes a Day

(6) Get Off "Automatic Pilot"

(11) Develop a Bedtime Ritual

(13) Practice Mindfulness

(15) Pick Up a Pen

(17) Schedule Your Priorities

(20) Do One Big Thing Daily

(28) Practice More Recovery Tools

(29) Train Your Brain

(30) Focus

(36) Be ADD No More!

(39) Hit the Pause Button At Least Twice a Day

(45) Stick to Your Schedule

(47) Use Caffeine Wisely

(49) Use Apps for Health and Vitality

(55) Add Yoga or Pilates

(61) Conquer Jet Lag

(70) Schedule a Standing Meal with a Friend

Appendix 3

Resources to Help with Your Simple Changes

Apps

Deep breathing and Meditation

- Pocket Meditation
- BreatheX
- BreatheToRelax
- BreatheBuddy
- Relax & Rest

Dietary

- MyNetDiary
- MyPlate by Livestrong
- NutritionMenu

Brain Training

- Lumosity
- CogniFit Brain Fitness

- Brain Trainer Special
- Brain Fitness Pro
- Fit Brains Trainer
- Eidetic- Learn & Remember

Exercise

- Cardiograph
- MyFitnessPal
- Yoga Studio (core)
- Pocket Yoga(core)
- Daily Ab Workout (core)
- Instant Fitness (core)
- Learn Pilates (core)
- Boot Camp Challenge
- Teemo: the fitness adventure game!
- Map My Fitness+ Workout Trainer
- Zombies, Run!
- Walk Tracker Pro
- Trails
- Tempo Magic Pro
- Strava Cycling

Websites

- **V2 Performance:** www.V2performance.com. My own website, with information and a video of the Exercises for Simple Changes.
- **Academy of Nutrition and Dietetics (formerly American Dietetic Association):** http://www.eatright.org
- **American Council on Fitness:** www.acefitness.org
- **American Diabetes Association:** www.diabetes.org

- **American Heart Association:** http://www.heart.org
- **National Institutes of Health:** http://www.nih.gov/

Books

- Kevin Cashman. *The Pause Principle: Step Back to Lead Forward.* Berrett-Koehler Publishers. 2012.

- Chris Crowley & Henry S. Lodge. *Younger Next Year: Live Strong, Fit, and Sexy—Until You're 80 and Beyond.* Workman Publishing, 1st reprint edition. 2007.

- Charles Duhigg. *The Power of Habit: Why We Do What We Do In Life and Business.* Random House, NY. 2014

- Daniel Goleman. *Focus, The Hidden Driver of Excellence.* Harper Collins. 2013

- Heidi Grant Halvorson. *Succeed: How We Can Reach Our Goals.* Plume, reprint edition. 2011.

- Bill Kovach & Tom Rosensteil. *Blur: How to Know What's True in the Age of Information Overload.* Bloomsbury USA; Reprint edition. 2011

Cookbooks

- *The Essential Eating Well Cookbook* by Patsy Jamieson, 2006.

- *Weeknight Wonders: Delicious, Healthy Dinners in 30 Minutes or Less* by Ellie Krieger, RD

- *Week in a Day* by Rachel Ray (Not always healthy choices but easy)

- *Beating the Lunch Box Blues: Fresh Ideas for Lunches on the Go!* by J.M. Hirsch and Rachel Ray

- *Spices of Life: Simple and Delicious Recipes for Great Health* by Nina Simonds, Knopf, 2005.

- *The America's Test Kitchen Healthy Family Cookbook* by the editors at America's Test Kitchen, America's Test Kitchen, 2010.

- *The Santa Monica Farmers' Market Cookbook: Seasonal Foods, Simple Recipes, and Stories from the Market and Farm* by Amelia Saltsman, 2007.

- *The New American Heart Association Cookbook, 8th Edition* by American Heart Association

- *Fit Food - Eating Well for Life* by Ellen Haas, 2005.

- *American Dietetic Association Cooking Healthy Across America* edited by Kristine Napier, 2005.

- *5 a Day: The Better Health Cookbook* by Elizabeth Pivonka and Barbara Berry, 2002.

Appendix 4

The Yerkes-Dodson Law

As this diagram shows, stress (termed "Arousal") improves performance if the stress is appropriate to the task. However, if the stress is too high or goes on for too long, it weakens performance.

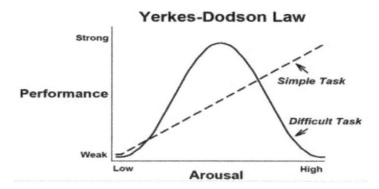

Diamond, David M. Cognitive, Endocrine and Mechanistic Perspectives on Non-Linear Relationships Between Arousal and Brain Function. Dose-Response: An International Journal. Jan 2005; 3(1): 1–7. http://www.ncbi.nlm.nih.gov/pmc/articles/PMC2657838/; Yerkes R.M., Dodson J.D. The relation of strength of stimulus to rapidity of habit-formation. J.Comp.Neurol.Psychol. 1908;18:459–482

Appendix 5

Exercises for Simple Changes

Here is a very brief 10-20 minute strength and flexibility program. It is meant to be very simple and can be added upon later. If you would like to see a video of this workout along with some breathing exercises go to www.v2performance.com/.

Also, before you start any new exercise program, be sure to see a qualified healthcare provider. These exercises are suggestions only: Don't substitute them for medical diagnosis or treatment. Do these at your own risk and stop if you feel pain, become faint, or experience shortness of breath.

For full color copies of this program and a step by step video go to http://v2performance.com/exercise-programs/

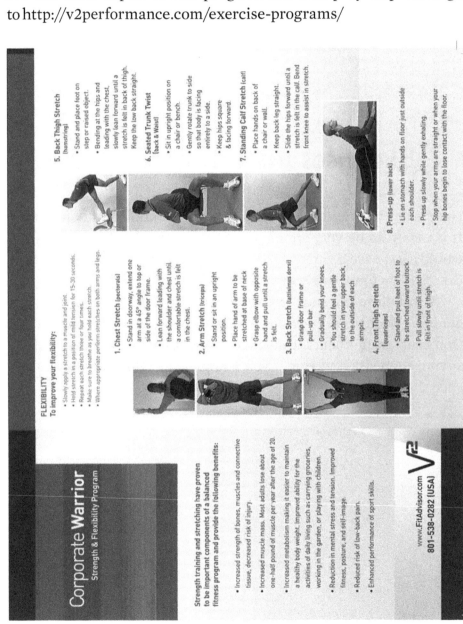

Corporate Warrior
Strength & Flexibility Program

Strength training and stretching have proven to be important components of a balanced fitness program and provide the following benefits:

• Increased strength of bones, muscles and connective tissue, decreased risk of injury.

• Increased muscle mass. Most adults lose about one-half pound of muscle per year after the age of 20.

• Increased metabolism making it easier to maintain a healthy body weight. Improved ability for the activities of daily living such as carrying groceries, working in the garden, or playing with children.

• Reduction in mental stress and tension. Improved fitness, posture, and self-image.

• Reduced risk of low-back pain.

• Enhanced performance of sport skills.

www.FitAdvisor.com
801-538-0282 (USA)

FLEXIBILITY
To improve your flexibility:

• Slowly apply a stretch to a muscle and joint.

• Hold stretch in a position of mild tension for 15-30 seconds.

• Repeat each stretch three or four times.

• Make sure to breathe as you hold each stretch.

• Where appropriate perform stretches on both arms and legs.

1. Chest Stretch (pectoralis)

• Stand in doorway, extend one arm at a 45° angle to top or side of the door frame.

• Lean forward leading with the shoulder and chest until a comfortable stretch is felt in the chest.

2. Arm Stretch (triceps)

• Stand or sit in an upright position.

• Place hand of arm to be stretched at base of neck

• Grasp elbow with opposite hand and pull until a stretch is felt.

3. Back Stretch (lattisimus dorsi)

• Grasp door frame or pull-up bar

• Gradually bend your knees.

• You should feel a gentle stretch in your upper back, to the outside of each armpit.

4. Front Thigh Stretch (quadriceps)

• Stand and pull heel of foot to be stretched toward buttock.

• Pull slowly until stretch is felt in front of thigh.

5. Back Thigh Stretch (hamstring)

• Stand and place foot on step or raised object.

• Bending at the hips and leading with the chest, slowly lean forward until a stretch is felt in back of thigh. Keep the low back straight.

6. Seated Trunk Twist (back & Waist)

• Sit in upright position on a chair or bench.

• Gently rotate trunk to side so that body is facing entirely to a side.

• Keep hips square & facing forward.

7. Standing Calf Stretch (calf)

• Place hands on back of a chair or wall.

• Keep back leg straight.

• Slide the hips forward until a stretch is felt in the calf. Bend front knee to assist in stretch.

8. Press-up (lower back)

• Lie on stomach with hands on floor just outside each shoulder.

• Press up slowly while gently exhaling.

• Stop when your arms are straight or when your hip bones begin to lose contact with the floor.

STRENGTH TRAINING

While strength training, complete one set of 12-15 repetitions, working the muscle to the point of fatigue. Breathe normally throughout the exercises.

Using the Door Attachment

- Always anchor along the hinge side of the door. Make sure the door is securely locked. TEST TO MAKE SURE BAND IS SECURE BEFORE BEGINNING!

1. Chest Press (pectorals)

- Anchor tube at shoulder height.
- Start movement with palms forward, elbows out, hands near shoulders.
- Press forward, to near full extension.

2. Standing Row (upper back)

- Keep tube anchored at chest height.
- Stand far enough back from door so arms can be fully extended, palms facing each other.
- Squeeze shoulder blades together and pull elbows back parallel to shoulders.

3. Triceps Pressdown (back of arm)

- Anchor tube over the top of the door.
- Grasp tube handles with forearms slightly above parallel to the floor.
- Holding elbows close to sides press down until elbows are almost straight.

4. Squat (quads, gluteals, hamstrings)

- Place tube under feet, shoulder width apart and knees bent.
- With tube behind arms grasp handles, palms forward at shoulder level.
- Straighten legs to standing.

5. Military Press (shoulders)

- Place tube under feet, shoulder width apart and knees slightly bent.
- With tube behind arms grasp handles, palms forward at shoulder level.
- Press up to nearly straight arms.

6. Biceps Curls (front of arms)

- Place tube under feet, shoulder width apart and knees slightly bent.
- Grasp tube with arms straight, palms forward.
- Pull arms toward chest until they are at shoulder height.

7. Hip Adduction (inner thigh)

- Anchor "figure 8" shaped tube securely at floor level.
- Stand with side of body facing anchor point.
- Place foot nearest the anchor through tube with feet slightly apart.
- Move inner foot over outer foot using a chair for support.

8. Hip Abduction (outer thigh)

- Anchor "figure 8" shaped tube securely at floor level.
- Stand with side of body facing anchor point.
- Place foot furthest from anchor through tube with feet slightly apart.
- Move foot to the outside away from anchor point, using a chair for support.

9. Prone Extension (lower back)

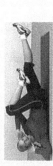

- Lie face down with arms & legs extended.
- Lift opposite arm and leg slightly off the ground (i.e. right arm, left leg).
- Hold for 3 counts, lower slowly, and alternate sides.
- Keep hips in contact with floor at all times. Do not arch back.

10. Combo Crunch (middle and side abdominals)

- Lie on back, feet flat on floor, knees bent.
- For middle abs, press lower back into floor, raising shoulders off floor.
- For outside abs, move shoulder toward opposite knee, repeat for opposite side.

References

1. The Mind Unleashed. 11 Reasons Dehydration Is Making You Sick And Fat. 8 September, 2014 at 00:11. http://themindunleashed. org/2014/09/11-reasons-dehydration-making-sick-fat.html

2. Institute of Medicine of the National Academies. Dietary Reference Intakes: Water, Potassium, Sodium, Chloride, and Sulfate. February 11, 2004. http://www.iom.edu/Reports/2004/ Dietary-Reference-Intakes-Water-Potassium-Sodium-Chloride-and-Sulfate.aspx.

3. Department of Health and Human Services. 2008 Physical Activity Guidelines for Americans. 2008. www.health.gov/ paguidelines/guidelines/#pag

4. Schmidt, W.D., Biwer, C.J., & Kalscheuer. Effects of Long versus short Bout Exercise on Fitness and Weight Loss in Overweight Females. Journal of the American College of Nutrition. 2001, Vol 20, Issue 5, pp 494-501, DOI: 10.1080/07315724.2001.10719058

5. About.com Psychology: http://psychology.about.com/od/yindex/ f/yerkes-dodson-law.htm; Diamond, David M. Cognitive, Endocrine and Mechanistic Perspectives on Non-Linear Relationships Between Arousal and Brain Function. Dose-Response: An International Journal. Jan 2005; 3(1): 1–7. http://www.ncbi.nlm.nih.gov/pmc/ articles/PMC2657838/; Yerkes R.M., Dodson J.D. The relation of

strength of stimulus to rapidity of habit-formation. J.Comp.Neurol. Psychol. 1908;18:459–482

6.   New York Times Anxiety In-Depth Report
http://www.nytimes.com/health/guides/symptoms/stress-and-anxiety/print.html?module=Search&mabReward=relbias%3Aw%2C%7B%222%22%3A%22RI%3A14%22%7D

7.   Online World Observer. How a bad night's sleep could age your brain by five YEARS: Poor quality slumber causes loss of memory and concentration. MAY 11, 2014 2:52 PM
http://worldobserveronline.com/2014/05/11/bad-nights-sleep-age-brain-five-years-poor-quality-slumber-causes-loss-memory-concentration/

8.   Alhola P, Polo-Kantola P. Sleep deprivation: Impact on cognitive performance.
Neuropsychiatr Dis Treat. 2007;3(5):553-67. PMID:19300585 http://www.ncbi.nlm.nih.gov/pubmed/19300585.

9.   National Sleep Foundation. Seven Things You Need to Know About Excessive Sleepiness. http://sleepfoundation.org/sleep-news/seven-things-you-need-know-about-excessive-sleepiness.

10.   Nedergaard, Maiken. Et al. Sleep Drives Metabolite Clearance from the Adult Brain.
Science 18 October 2013: Vol. 342 no. 6156 pp. 373-377 . DOI: 10.1126/science.1241224. http://www.sciencemag.org/content/342/6156/373.

11.   Harvard Health Publications. Blue Light has a dark side. MAY 2012.
http://www.health.harvard.edu/newsletters/Harvard_Health_Letter/2012/May/blue-light-has-a-dark-side.

12. Hollis et al (2008). Weight loss during intensive intervention phase of the weight-loss maintenance trial. American Journal of Preventative Medicine. Vol 35 Iss 2 pp 118-126 DOI: 10.1016/j.amepre.2008.04.013

13. Wilmot, E.G., et. al. Sedentary time in adults and the association with diabetes, cardiovascular disease and death: systematic review and meta-analysis. Diabetologia. November 2012, Volume 55, Issue 11, pp 2895-2905. http://link.springer.com/article/10.1007/s00125-012-2677-z Diabetologia.

14. Reynolds, Gretchen. The New York Times: Well. October 17, 2012, 12:01 a.m. http://well.blogs.nytimes.com/2012/10/17/get-up-get-out-dont-sit/

15. Covey, Stephen R. *The 7 Habits of Highly Effective People: Powerful Lessons in Personal Change.* 1990. Simon Schuster Ltd. UK. 326. p. 161.

16. Schwartz, Tony. The 90-Minute Solution: How Building in Periods of Renewal Can Change Your Work and Your Life. 05/18/2010 8:51 am EDT Updated: 11/17/2011 9:02 am EST. http://www.huffingtonpost.com/tony-schwartz/work-life-balance-the-90_b_578671.html.

17. Lerche Davis, Jeanie. WebMD feature. 5 Ways Pets Can Improve Your Health.
http://www.webmd.com/hypertension-high-blood-pressure/features/health-benefits-of-pets.

18. Sullivan, Bob and Thompson, Hugh. Brain, Interrupted. May 3, 2013. *http:/Sulliv/www.nytimes.com/2013/05/05/opinion/sunday/a-focus-on-distraction.html?_r=0*

19. Rock, David. Your Brain at Work. Easily distracted: why it's hard to focus, and what to do about it. October 4, 2009. http://www.psychologytoday.com/blog/your-brain-work/200910/easily-distracted-why-its-hard-focus-and-what-do-about-it.

20. Chow, Denise. Why Humans Are Bad at Multitasking. June 13, 2013 12:46pm ET. http://www.livescience.com/37420-multitasking-brain-psychology.html

21. Hollis et al (2008). Weight loss during intensive intervention phase of the weight-loss maintenance trial. American Journal of Preventative Medicine. Vol 35 Iss 2 pp 118-126 DOI: 10.1016/j.amepre.2008.04.013

22. Wansink, B. & Van Ittersum, K. Portion Size Me: Downsizing Our Consumption Norms. Journal of the American Dietetic Association. 2007. Vol 107 Issue 7 pp 1103-1106 http://mindlesseating.org/lastsupper/pdf/portion_size_me_JADA_2007.pdf

23. CDC. Overweight and Obesity. www.cdc.gov/obesity/data/prevalence-maps.html

24. Wansink, B. & Roizen, M. Mindless Dieting. Newsletter #1 of a Series. mindlesseating.org/pdf/mindless_dieting_01.pdf

25. Brian Wansink and Katherine Abowd Johnson. (2014) The Clean Plate Club: About 92% of Self-Served Food is Eaten. The International Journal of Obesity, doi: 10.1038/ijo.2014.104

26. Wilmot, EG Sedentary time in adults and the association with diabetes, cardiovascular disease and death: systematic review and meta-analysis.

27. Ruxton, Carrie. (2009). Health aspects of caffeine: benefits and risks. Nursing Standard, 24(9), 41–48.

28. Alpert, Patricia T. The Health Lowdown on Caffeine. Home Health Care Management & Practice. Published online before print February 6, 2012, doi: 10.1177/1084822311435543. June 2012. vol. 24 no. 3. Pp. 156–158.

29. National Sleep Foundation. What Causes Insomnia? http://sleepfoundation.org/sleep-disorders-problems/insomnia/causes.

30. Barnett, Jeffrey E. Shale, Allison J. Alternative techniques. April 2013, Vol 44, No. 4 Print version: page 48. http://www.apa.org/monitor/2013/04/ce-corner.aspx

31. WebMD. Health & Balance. What Is Holistic Medicine? http://www.webmd.com/balance/guide/what-is-holistic-medicine

32. American Heart Association. Sugar 101. Updated Feb. 24, 2014 http://www.heart.org/HEARTORG/GettingHealthy/NutritionCenter/HealthyEating/Sugar—101_UCM_306024_Article.jsp.

33. National Institute on Aging. Can We Prevent Aging? http://www.nia.nih.gov/health/publication/can-we-prevent-aging.

34. Gahche, J. et. Al. (2011). Dietary Supplement Use Among U.S. Adults Has Increased Since NHANES III (1998-1994). NCHS Data Brief. http://www.cdc.gov/nchs/data/databriefs/db61.pdf

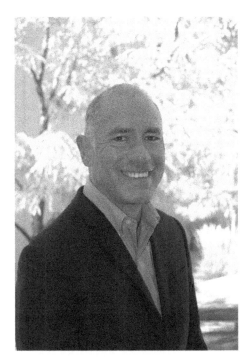

Gregory Florez has been changing people's lives for 28 years. He is the founder and CEO of V2 Performance.com, an international consulting and training firm. Gregory is an internationally known speaker, facilitator, and coach who works with Global 1000 companies, teams, and individuals to increase their vitality in our high velocity world. He also coaches individuals to help them make Simple Changes in their lives to increase their happiness, energy, and vitality. Gregory lives in Salt Lake City with his wife Kerry and strives to keep a balance of vitality/velocity in his own life. He can be contacted at www.v2performance.com regarding training and coaching.